T5-AGU-151

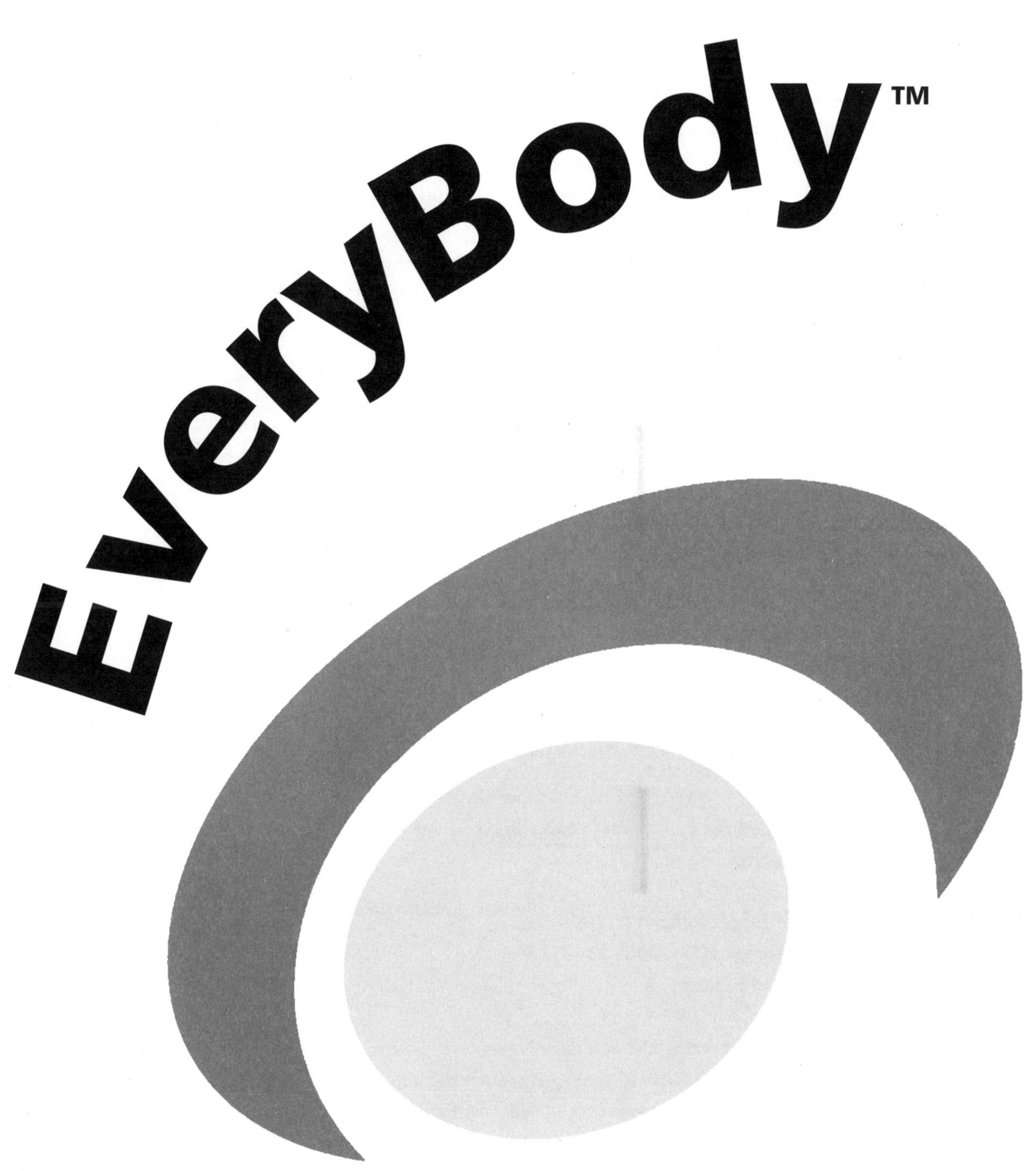

Preventing HIV and Other Sexually Transmitted Diseases Among Young Teens

Revised Edition

Deborah Schoeberlein

RAD Educational Programs
Carbondale, Colorado

RAD Educational Programs

(Redefining Actions & Decisions)

provides a unique, interactive educational approach to the promotion of healthy human development based on direct and compassionate communication with youths and adults. RAD develops specialized educational materials, and presents program implementation and technical support services. RAD offers professional development training to assist teachers and other professionals in implementing EveryBody™.

Published by: RAD Educational Programs
PO Box 1433
Carbondale, CO 81623

First Printing 2000
Second Printing 2001, Revised Edition

Printed in the United States of America

Publisher's Cataloging-in-Publication Data

Schoeberlein, Deborah R.
EveryBody : Preventing HIV and other sexually transmitted diseases among young teens / Deborah Schoeberlein. -- 2nd ed.
p. cm.
Includes bibliographical references.
Preassigned LCCN: 2001 130232
ISBN: 0-9679256-1-4

1. Sexually transmitted diseases--Prevention--Study and teaching. 2. AIDS (Disease)--Prevention--Study and teaching. 3. Health education. 4. Sex instruction for teenagers. I. Title.

RA644.V4S36 2001 613.9'51'071
QB101-200309

10 9 8 7 6 5 4 3 2

Contents

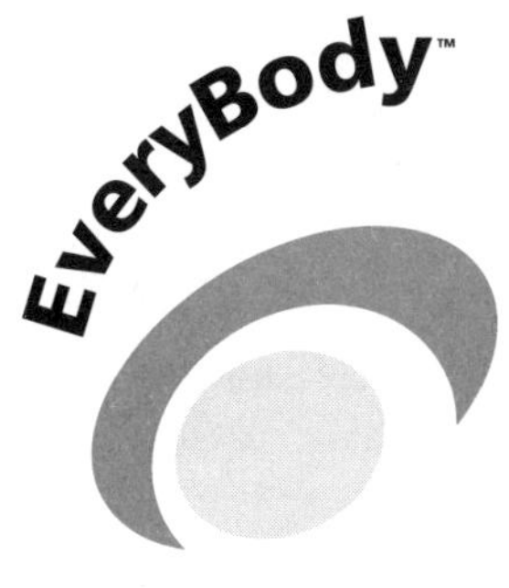

continued on back of this page

Beyond *Just Say No*

A year ago RAD first published *EveryBody*™. Now RAD is pleased to present the revised edition of this book. In the time between I have been talking about *EveryBody* instead of writing it. And I have been working with and listening to many people across America using the curriculum.

There is reason to believe that an enlightened educational approach prevents new HIV infections and other sexually transmitted diseases (STDs). In many communities, the commitment to HIV/STD prevention continues to grow. Condom use increases as young people support the norm of using protection. Furthermore, a strong sense of hope prevails that sophisticated medical strategies may soon slow or even stop the AIDS epidemic. In addition, more and more youth are choosing to wait longer before engaging in the behaviors that pose a risk of HIV/STD infection. We have much to be grateful for.

Despite these important gains, there is also cause for concern. In too many places, interest in and commitment to HIV education have diminished even though the rates of new HIV infections remain constant in the United States and the AIDS epidemic expands worldwide. Complacency grows as people count on the future appearance of wonder drugs to solve the AIDS problem. Religious, moral and political visions increasingly affect government funding and school district policy on health education. As a result, "abstinence-only" curricula are gaining ground despite their lack of efficacy and "abstinence-based" curricula are often subject to attack.

In these unsettling times, teachers need to be reassured that "abstinence-based" curricula such as *EveryBody* are of critical importance for adolescent students. Teachers also need confidence that such curricula are effective, developmentally appropriate and academically sound. Finally, teachers need support for health education and HIV/STD prevention from members of their school community, including administrators, parents, community members and, most importantly, students.

I believe that an "abstinence-only" approach at the middle school level has proven irresponsible from an educational and public health perspective. Young teens can — and must — learn to handle the far more responsible message that there are two ways to prevent HIV and other STDs: **you can avoid all behaviors that pose a risk (risk elimination) or you can make those behaviors less risky (risk reduction).**

From the parental perspective, children in today's world have both more to learn and more to lose than ever before. Whereas schools teach public health, parents still bear the responsibility for communicating family beliefs and values regarding HIV/STD prevention. Unfortunately, many parents hesitate to address these issues perhaps unaware that their contribution is far more powerful than that of any school.

Today's health professionals also face challenges in encouraging HIV/STD prevention among adolescents. Health care providers have more concerns to address and more care to give than ever before. However, they also have less time to spend with their teenage patients. Regrettably, this situation exists at a time when HIV and other STDs seriously threaten teens' present and future health. For many young women, the consequences of unprotected sexual behaviors can impair future fertility. Then, too, incurable though not lethal STDs impact significantly on general health and well-being. And of course, HIV continues to kill.

With the revised edition of *EveryBody,* RAD hopes to further accentuate its original approach to HIV/STD education at the middle school level. I hope that the points listed below give you — teachers, parents, health professionals — a sense of new direction and renewed energy for the part you can play in disease prevention.

As HIV/STD Educators, We Can:

- Teach disease prevention in context with the deeper issues of how kids live their lives. Prevention is fundamentally about communication, healthy choices, responsible behaviors and self-awareness.
- Present "abstinence-based" HIV/STD education. The only way to slow and ultimately stop AIDS is by educating youth about risk elimination and risk reduction. There is no mixed message here; both options can prevent HIV and other STDs.
- Focus on the links between sex and drugs. Discussion of cause and effect reveal that disease prevention and drug prevention go hand in hand.

continued

- Integrate disease prevention into related courses such as Sex Education, Drug Prevention Programming or Character Education. Respect, responsibility, honesty, ethical behavior and healthy decision-making are common themes across curricula.
- Teach to standards and be accountable. Students need a variety of opportunities to internalize, personalize and demonstrate mastery of disease prevention messages. Presenting the curriculum is not enough; success is measured by the degree to which students adopt *EveryBody*'s wisdom.
- Recognize that risk taking is a normal and necessary part of adolescent development. The goal is to encourage exploration while discouraging (self) destructive actions. Teens need to take risks. They also need to distinguish between invigorating risks and debilitating ones.
- Identify the role of fear. Healthy fear is a normal and appropriate response to danger. Unhealthy fear can lead to phobias, paranoia and discrimination against people with HIV infection. Unhealthy fear is just that — unhealthy.
- Acknowledge feelings of anger. Youth have the right to be angry about the AIDS epidemic. However, it is important to recognize the potential for danger when anger controls actions. We can help teens transform their anger into energy for living.
- Examine our own personal beliefs about HIV and other STDs. As teachers and health care providers, we must separate our personal views from our professional responsibilities. Youth trust us to provide accurate information and nonjudgmental guidance. As parents, our charge is the opposite: we must share, strengthen and protect the beliefs our families hold dear.

New Mission

We live in the time of AIDS and other sexually transmitted diseases. The good news is that people with HIV, other STDs and AIDS are living longer and healthier lives that ever before. But, some teens are already quite ill, and others will get sick much too early and die before their time. Grief is a normal and necessary response to this situation.

It is also important to have hope. We live in an age of increased understanding about human behavior. We recognize that "just say no" simply does not work. Instead, the dual option approach to HIV/STD prevention makes behavioral sense. However, we must teach young people about the necessity of mature decisions at a time when their brains are not yet fully developed. Rather than having us expect kids to be wise before their time, the dual option approach helps us assist them in controlling their impulses and accessing real consequences while physiologically immature.

EveryBody cannot provide all the answers. But it does teach youth about self-awareness, healthy decision-making and responsibility. It also models compassion. Kids need guidance. Young adults need skills. And we — their teachers, parents and health care providers — need expertise, patience and all the help we can get from one another.

Perseverance is essential, as is courage. Do not judge the success of HIV/STD education by immediate changes in teens' activities since behaviors evolve over time. Likewise, do not assume failure should some kids seem to reject your efforts. Instead, do your best to believe that you can make an enduring difference for young people after they leave your classroom, home or clinic.

You set forth on a mission to focus on the real challenges of living, because it is in this *realistic* realm that we can make our greatest contribution to society. HIV/STD prevention is up to everybody. Our children, and the world they inherit, depend on it.

Deborah Schoeberlein
March 2001

Introduction to EveryBody

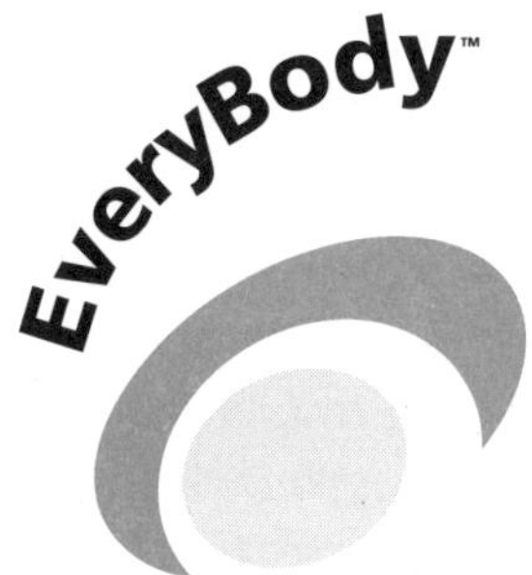

HIV and sexually transmitted disease (STD) prevention is fundamentally a matter of communication between people. Of course, prevention begins with the individual and includes education and self-awareness. But just as these diseases are transmitted from person to person, the process of prevention occurs between people. Humans are social creatures. HIV and other STDs are human diseases. The challenges they pose are unique to us.

The AIDS epidemic has transformed people's lives and made unlikely experts out of many individuals affected by HIV and its related issues. A tiny virus, HIV became a huge public health concern by the late 1980s. Its toll in terms of human tragedy continues to rise and with it a growing need for research, health care, and prevention. In response, many of us *learned by doing* — by necessity, we became AIDS advocates and caregivers, policy makers and educators. Then as now, we do work in the AIDS field because the work has to be done.

Without a cure or vaccine for HIV, prevention is still the most effective way to slow, and perhaps, stop the AIDS epidemic. Although the basic points of HIV prevention are fairly straightforward, the process of translating knowledge into safe(r) behavior is incredibly complicated. To be effective, HIV education must address some of the most intimate aspects of personal experience and activity. In addition to the behavioral issues, the political challenges to successful programming are formidable and include the current push towards abstinence-only curricula. Presenting HIV education, like participating in it, can be awkward and even difficult. Ignoring HIV education, however, can be lethal.

I began teaching about HIV prevention in 1989 as an Outward Bound instructor. My students posed basic questions about AIDS and much more complex questions about how HIV would affect their lives. In 1992, I founded a nonprofit organization called Redefining Actions and Decisions (RAD) Educational Programs expressly for the purpose of developing and implementing interactive HIV education. Since 1992, RAD has expanded from a grassroots program serving 2,500 fifth-twelfth grade students a semester in the Colorado mountains to a national program meeting the needs of students across America through general distribution of EveryBody™ which is now the featured curriculum of a 5-year federally funded national dissemination project.

I believe that HIV prevention requires a radical approach — we need education that is compassionate and flexible, explicit and honest, direct and ambitious. We need to address prevention in the real world and we need to apply the rigors of scientific research to our work. Most of all we need to develop and use HIV education techniques that are effective and relevant for contemporary youth.

EveryBody activities are unusual and, in many ways, radical. I designed these activities in the classroom and modified them over time to meet the needs of students as well as their teachers and families. In some ways, I wrote the curriculum backwards — I started with youths' questions and comments, applied common sense and my familiarity with experiential education, and found out later how the activities were connected to scientific theory. As I learned more about health education and prevention, I sought input from many people representing different scientific and educational disciplines. As a result, the curriculum grew stronger, deeper and more flexible over time.

In 1996, the Elizabeth Glaser Pediatric AIDS Foundation generously gave RAD funding to conduct a 21-month national demonstration project. The aim of this project was to learn if regular classroom teachers could successfully implement the RAD model in diverse middle schools from four states. Charles Deutsch, Sc.D., of the Harvard School of Public Health and John Brett, Ph.D., from the University of Colorado at Denver were the principal investigators for the independent evaluation that accompanied this project. The resulting quantitative and qualitative data showed significant positive impacts on students' knowledge, perceptions, and attitudes about HIV, AIDS prevention, and personal risk-taking [1]. Students demonstrated significant gains in comfort with talking to peers and teachers about HIV prevention. Also, at a time when young teens often increase risky behaviors, students in this study maintained low levels of actual and intended risky behaviors from baseline through three-month posttest. In addition, students, teachers, administrators, parents, and other community members strongly supported the curriculum. In other words, the research showed that EveryBody works: *it is memorable, durable and portable* [2].

As its name implies, EveryBody *is for everybody*: teachers, families, health professionals, others who work with youth, and most importantly young teens, themselves. Above all, EveryBody is about helping adolescents develop the habits of being informed regarding their own health and being responsible for preventing HIV and other STDs. Some adults may feel that EveryBody goes beyond what is expected for a fifth through ninth grade curriculum. However, EveryBody is developmentally appropriate and the research shows that it matches the needs of today's youths. EveryBody targets young teens, many of whom have not initiated risky behaviors, with the objective of providing a prevention paradigm to help students shape their future activities. EveryBody also provides potentially life-saving content for those youth already at risk for HIV and other STDs.

EveryBody has a very specific mission: to facilitate communication about HIV/STD prevention and to promote safe(r) behaviors among young teens. EveryBody does not seek or claim to do everything that comprehensive health education can and must do. In the context of HIV/STD education, EveryBody does touch on alcohol and drug prevention and the impact of the media. But, the curriculum does not focus on these areas. Furthermore, EveryBody assumes that students, teachers, and other adults have some familiarity with basic communication skills. If needed, I urge the reader to seek out additional resources to supplement EveryBody.

With the publication of this book, I now turn my attention toward supporting teachers, families, health professionals and others as they use EveryBody to promote HIV/STD prevention among youth. RAD continues to offer professional development training in EveryBody. In addition, our interactive website **www.preventaids.net** provides an online opportunity for dialogue about HIV/STD education and the process of implementing EveryBody.

EveryBody is not a static curriculum. It should be used, adapted, and enhanced. It is a bit like the bones that stabilize our bodies — EveryBody provides a solid structure that can support a unique and valuable individual with particular experiences and needs. You, the reader and the user, are empowered to make this curriculum your own. It is a living curriculum, and it celebrates life.

1. Brett, J., et al., Student Responses to an Explicit Middle School HIV/AIDS Education Program in Conservative Communities. in review.
2. Brett, J., et al., The Fernwood Project: Final Report on Statistical Data. 1998, Denver, CO: University of Colorado.

Overview of EveryBody™

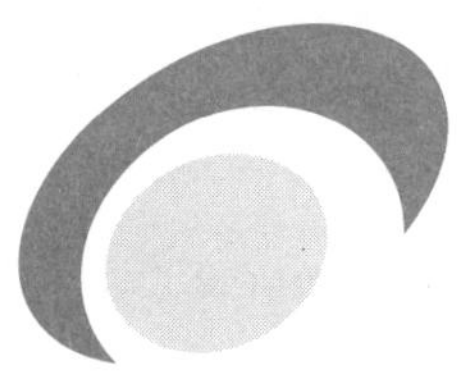

Fifth through ninth grade students are fascinating, intense, often challenging, and remarkably resilient. They can be the most curious of learners and the most patient of teachers. They can develop and articulate a keen awareness of the tensions that exist between childhood and adulthood.

EveryBody celebrates early adolescence as a valid and necessary passage; a time of extraordinary growth. The curriculum affirms the premise that informed skillful adolescents are capable of making healthy decisions to prevent HIV and other STDs. EveryBody honors young adolescents' capacity for learning and exploration; it strengthens communication skills and decision making by building on developmentally appropriate activities and learning experiences.

EveryBody fosters active learning. Its flexible format is responsive to the wide variation in youths' cognitive and emotional maturity, life experience, and resiliency factors. EveryBody explores the boundaries between thinking and doing, perceiving and knowing.

Interactive, experiential learning techniques engage youth and adults in educational activities that are structured yet spontaneous, and above all safe. EveryBody provides accurate health information in a manner respectful of students' personal beliefs and family norms. EveryBody activities guide teachers to separate their personal beliefs from professional responsibilities. The protections and limitations of confidentiality are recognized and discussed in the classroom.

EveryBody activities offer a safe proxy for actual real life experience. Students learn, practice and internalize potentially life-saving knowledge, attitudes, skills and behaviors. The behaviors that place people at risk for HIV/STD infection are primarily social. Likewise, HIV/STD education and healthy behaviors take place within relationships. In EveryBody, prevention of these diseases is directly linked to communication and human connection, personal rights as well as public responsibility.

EveryBody's Approach to Risky Behaviors

EveryBody incorporates current research on adolescent development. For most teens, a positive and productive adolescence is characterized, in part, by normal, healthy risk-taking experiences [1]. EveryBody rejects the categorization of teenagers as a "high-risk group." Rather than interpret teens' risky behaviors as evidence of adolescent invincibility, EveryBody proposes that such behaviors often result from the combination of immature abstract reasoning and a lack of real life experience. Consequently, EveryBody strengthens young adolescents' understanding of options, actions, and potential outcomes.

EveryBody meets students where they are. It is relevant, engaging, and practical. It pertains to students' reality. Simple admonitions to avoid risks are developmentally inappropriate. Young adolescents need to know *why, how*, and *when* to protect themselves. Regrettably, HIV, AIDS and other STDs can extract a horrendously high price for learning done by trial and error.

EveryBody is an abstinence-based approach that promotes risk elimination as the safest way to prevent HIV/STD infections and also endorses risk reduction as an important component of HIV/STD prevention strategies. Lessons and activities promote the development, internalization, and actual use of prevention-related skills and knowledge; commitment to lifelong health; self-efficacy; hope for the future; and courage.

EveryBody aims to prevent interconnected high-risk behaviors and encourage interconnected protective factors. Young adolescents are understood as more than the sum of their risk and resiliency factors. The curriculum focuses on the role of healthy self-esteem in addressing prevention strategies for individuals, community and society.

EveryBody acknowledges the complex behavioral implications for HIV/STD prevention: individuals must understand, internalize, and remain committed to safe(r) behaviors. Young adolescents know that the world is complicated. EveryBody affirms the experience of reality and provides practical, acceptable prevention strategies for youths.

The curriculum addresses relevant psychosocial issues such as the experience of fear and anger in the context of HIV/STD prevention.* Healthy fear can be a motivator for safe(r) behaviors. However, unhealthy fear can be destructive. EveryBody reduces fears related to ignorance and misunderstanding. This approach helps youth learn to identify, acknowledge, and transform the energy of fear into productive action or understanding.

In addition, EveryBody activities examine anger as an uncomfortable emotion and guide students to see that such emotions does not necessitate (self) destructive risk taking. Young adolescents are capable of understanding that people can feel anger about HIV and still be able to protect themselves.

Prevention Strategies

EveryBody focuses on high-risk behaviors as opposed to high-risk groups. In other words, *it's not who you are, but what you do that can put you at risk for HIV.* EveryBody explains the mechanism of risk for HIV/STD infection beyond listing specific risky behaviors. The likelihood of HIV/STD infection is described through an equation in which the riskiness of personal behaviors interacts with other variables such as the frequency of risky behaviors, the prevalence of HIV/STD in the community, underlying health status, access to care, and chance.

This curriculum addresses sexuality as a normal part of human experience. Sexual behaviors are discussed in clinical terms that are non-threatening and non-sensational. Activities include mention of the three highest risk sexual behaviors: vaginal, anal and oral intercourse. EveryBody does not endorse limiting this description as students may mistakenly assume that any behaviors not labeled *risky* are *safe.*

EveryBody presents two main prevention strategies: risk elimination and risk reduction. From a public health perspective, risk elimination represents true safety. Yet many people do not choose these safe options or cannot exercise their right to such a choice (as in cases of rape or trauma). Therefore, developmentally-appropriate discussion of risk reduction, including the subject of safer sex, is critical.

*HIV is an STD. However, the form HIV/STD is accepted as a shortened version of "HIV and other STDs."

Risk Elimination

Maintaining a lifestyle for an indeterminate period of time that does not include any behaviors that put you at risk of HIV/STD infection, including sexual intercourse (vaginal, oral and/or anal), use of alcohol or other illegal drugs, and any needle-sharing activities.

EveryBody uses the term "risk elimination" instead of "abstinence" given the common association between abstinence and religious or moral beliefs. Risk elimination is a more precise description of the desired behavioral outcome.

Risk Reduction

Using techniques that reduce the risk of disease transmission which include the use of effective barriers (such as latex condoms) as well as clean needles and injection drug paraphernalia.

Safe Sex

Sex within a mutually monogamous, trusting relationship between people who have tested negative for HIV and other STDs, don't share needles, and have no other risky behaviors. Typically, such relationships have a high level of mutual respect and communication.

Safer Sex

Sex involving use of risk reduction techniques. This type of sexual activity is safer than unprotected sex, but still contains some risk of disease transmission.

One of EveryBody's goals is for students to adopt risk elimination as an active choice and feel good about their choice. People have different expectations for how long they are willing to adopt risk elimination. EveryBody suggests that it is most important to focus on prevention in the present and immediate future. Staying healthy now is of the utmost importance, and sets precedence for future behavior.

EveryBody presents risk elimination as an investment in a person's future opportunities and choices. Safe sex is possible for healthy people. However, the option for safe sex can be jeopardized if one or both partners are infected with a transmissible disease.

EveryBody teaches about risk elimination from a positive perspective — emphasizing the benefits of eliminating risk rather than using scare tactics, i.e. "you'll die if you don't choose risk elimination."

EveryBody teaches that correct and consistent use of condoms can prevent transmission of HIV and STDs, but does **not** guarantee total safety. Condoms can fail. However, risk reduction can save lives and is a valid public health choice for sexually active people.

For some people, risk reduction is an intermediate step toward risk elimination. For others, risk reduction is a healthy way of life. In EveryBody, students create strategies to help them successfully use risk elimination or risk reduction strategies. Students practice making risk elimination and risk reduction statements, and developing plans to help them prevent HIV/STDs in real life situations.

1. Offer, D., K. Schoner-Reichl, and A. Boxer. Normal Adolescent Development: Empirical Research Findings, in Child and Adolescent Psychiatry, M. Lewis, Editor. 1996, Williams & Williams: Baltimore (MD). p. 278-290.

EveryBody™ in the Classroom

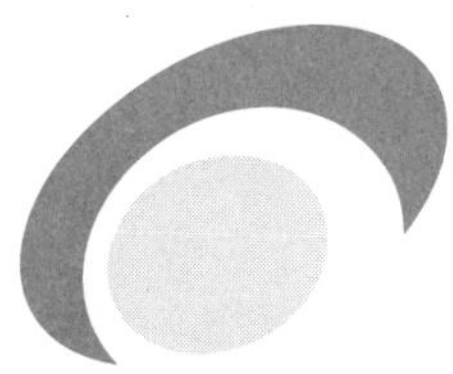

Successful HIV/STD education must be relevant and credible. Easy answers are rare, and complex dilemmas are the norm. Neither teacher nor students will know all the answers. Together, your students and you will reinforce the essential prevention messages and strengthen community norms that promote health.

HIV/STD education might not be personally relevant for every student in a single class. However, every student probably knows someone who could benefit from the prevention message. Teachers should encourage students to hear the information about HIV/STD prevention while honoring their own personal beliefs. Teachers are responsible for helping students reach their own healthy decisions using compassion and courage.

The classroom should be as comfortable as possible. The subject of HIV/STD prevention is uncomfortable for some students. Thus, a low stress, safe, physical space can enhance learning. EveryBody acknowledges that HIV/STD education is community information and prevention is a collective responsibility.

To establish a level of trust in the class and address concerns related to confidentiality, the class should develop a set of guidelines that includes statements regarding each person's right to his/her own opinions, allowing others to speak without interruption, and making no disrespectful or personal comments about other people. Such guidelines model the type of communication you want to foster in students' lives.

Teachers must be clear that they are presenting health information, not their own personal beliefs, religious views or values. During discussions, teachers must listen and respond professionally to direct statements or questions as well as the underlying issues which students' body language, voice, tone and/or word choice might suggest. Students commonly mask their real concerns and questions because of fear or embarrassment. Education about sexual issues and issues of death and dying can have a strong emotional impact on students.

References to illegal uses of drugs and alcohol should clearly state that these substances are illegal for students. EveryBody discourages students from using these substances (or have sex) by addressing the relationship between alcohol and other drug use and the risk of HIV/STD transmission.

Students often need time to adjust to non-traditional, interactive, modes of teaching. Teachers often put a lot of energy into the first part of experiential activities to compensate for students' initial reticence. A teacher's own discomfort can remind students of their concerns about HIV/STD education. Teachers need to remember that they are in control and aware of the big picture. In contrast, students are much more vulnerable.

Some people have strong responses to HIV/STD prevention education and may need to have private time away from the group. Teachers should give students permission to excuse themselves for time-out as needed. Encourage students to take care of themselves.

Different Approaches to EveryBody

EveryBody can be used as a comprehensive HIV/STD education curriculum, an enhancement program for existing health education, or a component of an integrated curriculum. EveryBody can be used with students in fifth through ninth grades organized in elementary, middle, junior high, or high schools. EveryBody can be used in non-school-based settings such as health clinics, after-school programs, youth centers, and camps. EveryBody is also a resource for parents and other family members seeking to provide HIV education for youth in the home.

Comprehensive Curriculum:

As organized in the recommended sequence, the combination of EveryBody activities and background information provides complete coverage of HIV/STD education content including: transmission, prevention, treatment, testing and psychosocial issues.

Enhancement Program:

EveryBody activities and background information can be used to supplement existing curriculum. EveryBody activities can also be substituted for less interactive, content specific, modules in other curricula.

Integrated Curriculum:

EveryBody is interdisciplinary and ideal for team teaching. It fosters cooperative and exploratory learning. The diversity of issues related to HIV/STD prevention is fascinating and well suited to student-driven learning.

HIV/STD education can be integrated easily into broad topics such as: public health, epidemics, personal behavior and public responsibility, science and the public, community organizing, discrimination, etc. The following bullets describe HIV/STD content areas that can be part of integrated curriculum for the middle grades:

- **Language Arts:** Poetry, fiction and non fiction about HIV, AIDS and other STDs; essays, other forms of creative writing, research papers and journal writing about HIV/STD-related issues; use of language in prevention education; analysis of the power of language and word choice: implicit and explicit meanings in vocabulary and terms; interview, reporting and presentation skills; analytical skills applied to movie reviews and/or book reports featuring stories about HIV or AIDS; etc.

- **Mathematics:** Data Analysis: reading and interpreting tables and graphs; probability: issues of likelihood of infection, prevalence within the population and other contributing factors to the probability of infection; compare & contrast statistics: analysis and calculations of positive and negative effects of the AIDS pandemic on populations; integers: ratios and proportions of regional prevalence to national and/or global statistics; variables: develop simple growth models utilizing data tables to find the rate of growth; graphing and charting; etc.

- **Science:** Scientific method; biology; human biology; microbiology; virology; sexually transmitted diseases; the human immune system; human reproduction; epidemics; epidemiology; population studies; HIV research; current ethical issues in HIV-related research; scientists involved with HIV-related research; etc.

- **Social Studies:** Prejudice and discrimination; historical responses to epidemics; legal issues and public health; morality and public health; cultural responses to illness; death and dying; implications of public education about personal behaviors; media messages about sexuality, risky behaviors and HIV/STD prevention; geography of the pandemic; biographies of the major contributors to the fight against HIV & AIDS; etc.

- **Visual and Performing Arts:** Full range of media to express perceptions, responses, messages and observations of HIV/STD-related issues; drama, music, and dance to educate about HIV and STDs from psychosocial issues to pure science; artistic expression of issues related to living with HIV or AIDS; artistic contributions of persons with HIV, AIDS and other significant illnesses; school participation in "A Day Without Art" in celebration of World AIDS Day; etc.

EveryBody within Coordinated School Health Programming

Good health and academic success go hand in hand. Students in schools with coordinated school health programs are likely to be well prepared for middle level HIV/STD education. They are also likely to receive ongoing reinforcement of prevention messages.

EveryBody has a role in coordinated school health programming. A common model for coordinated school health programs includes eight components [1]. Of these eight, EveryBody is directly connected to health education; health services; counseling, psychological and social services; as well as parent/community involvement. Indirectly, the other components of coordinated school health programming also pertain to HIV/STD-related issues.

EveryBody and Diversity Issues

EveryBody encourages educators and community members to tailor the activities to meet local norms and needs. There are common themes throughout the curriculum s uch as personal rights, public or community responsibility, safety, health, respect, and compassion. These themes are identified and treated as universal for a United States audience, although their application and interpretations may vary according to the specific ethnic, cultural, racial etc. composition of a community.

Customizing EveryBody

EveryBody is intended for local adaptation and school-based customization. However, the scope and sequence of the activities are most effective when implemented in the recommended sequences and enhanced by the chapters providing background information. The recommended activity sequences provide balanced coverage across three content categories: **Attitudes, Knowledge, and Skills.**

The recommended sequence for each grade level takes a minimum of several days to complete. The Lesson Extensions & Assessment activities vary in scope and length. The flexible format enables teachers to compress or expand their HIV/STD education unit as needed.

The recommended sequence might not match every student's needs and or every community's norms. In such cases, teachers can build a solid HIV/STD education unit by mixing-and-matching activities across grade levels. Many activities that are appropriate for several grade levels are recommended at one specific point in the sequence. If you create a customized sequence, coordinate your plans with other teachers in the school to prevent duplication and build a sequence that provides a balance of content categories.

Activity Format

An overview section begins each activity and provides the following information:

Content Categories: (Attitudes, Knowledge, and Skills)

Recommended grade level: (5-9)

Correlation to National Education Standards:
(Science Education (A-G) and Health Education (1-7)

Estimated Time excluding Lesson Extension & Assessment:
Ranges from 10 - 35 minutes per activity)

Materials (when required)

Set up (when required)

The body of each activity* includes the following sections:

Guiding Questions

Part 1 + (naturally occurring divisions in the lesson progressions)

Lesson Extension and Assessment

* The recommended sequences for grades 6-9 contain several activities that review information presented at younger grade levels. Be sure to pace the review process according to students' needs.

Assessment

The ultimate assessment of EveryBody's success is students' behavior outside of the classroom. However, several formal and informal activities can help teachers determine the extent to which students are learning and internalizing curricular content. The following topics are core elements of HIV/STD education at every grade level:

- **The life science of HIV, AIDS, and other STDs**
- **HIV/STD transmission**
- **HIV/STD prevention**
- **HIV antibody testing**
- **Psychosocial issues related to HIV/STDs**

The guiding questions that begin every activity establish what students should be able to answer by the end of the activity. Lesson extensions and assessment activities measure students' ability to respond to the guiding questions. The teacher can also observe students "in action" during those activities that involve students in small working groups.

Each EveryBody activity provides a section on Lesson Extensions & Assessment. The suggested assessment activities foster creativity, personalization of HIV/STD prevention messages, and development of communication skills. Students' performance should be linked to the overall quality of their work, the thoughtfulness of their responses, and the depth of their analysis.

(see next page for assessment criteria)

1. Marx, E., S.F. Wooley, and D.E. Northrop, Health is Academic: A Guide to Coordinated School Health Programs. 1998, New York: Teachers College Press.

The following chart identifies criteria a teacher might use to indicate students' advanced, proficient or unsatisfactory acquisition of key knowledge, attitudes and skills:

Advanced

1 Students' knowledge, attitudes and skills surpass the basic interpretation of relevant education standards.

2 Students provide accurate, thoughtful and in depth responses to the guiding questions for each activity.

3 Students demonstrate a high level of productive classroom participation, communication skills and performance in small groups.

4 Students demonstrate mastery of the content area as presented and are able to transfer the lessons from this content area into other arenas.

Proficient

1 Students' knowledge, attitudes and skills meet the basic interpretation of relevant education standards.

2 Students provide accurate, basic responses to the guiding questions presented for each activity.

3 Students demonstrate a basic level of productive classroom participation, communication skills and performance in small groups.

4 Students demonstrate mastery of the content area as presented.

Unsatisfactory

1 Students' knowledge, attitudes and skills fail to meet the basic interpretation of relevant education standards.

2 Students are unable to provide accurate, basic responses to the guiding questions presented for each activity.

3 Students demonstrate a minimal level of productive classroom participation, communication skills and performance in small groups.

4 Students have not mastered the content as presented.

Recommended Sequences for EveryBody™ Activities

5th Grade

The life science of HIV, AIDS, and other STDs

Introduce material from Information About HIV and AIDS
Cells, Bacteria and Viruses Activity

HIV/STD transmission

Doorways Activity

HIV/STD prevention

Gloves Activity
Talking About Condoms with Older Children
Bill of Rights and Responsibilities (Basic)

HIV antibody testing

Introduce material from Information About HIV and AIDS

Psychosocial issues related to HIV/STDs

Walk Like Activity

6th Grade

The life science of HIV, AIDS, and other STDs

Review material from Information About HIV and AIDS
HIV Replication Activity
HIV Mutation Activity

HIV/STD transmission

Review Doorways Activity

HIV/STD prevention

Review Talking About Condoms with Older Children
Review Bill of Rights and Responsibilities (Basic)

HIV antibody testing

Review material from Information About HIV and AIDS

Psychosocial issues related to HIV/STDs

Pennies Activity

7th Grade

The life science of HIV, AIDS, and other STDs

Review material from Information About HIV and AIDS

HIV/STD transmission

Review Doorways Activity

HIV/STD prevention

Talking About Condoms with Young Teens
Talking Risk Elimination and Risk Reduction
Review Bill of Rights and Responsibilities (Basic or Advanced)

HIV antibody testing

HIV Antibody Test Activity
Review material from Information About HIV and AIDS

Psychosocial issues related to HIV/STDs

Media Messages Discussion
It Could Happen to Me Activity

8th Grade

The life science of HIV, AIDS, and other STDs

Review material from Information About HIV and AIDS
STDs and Pregnancy Discussion
Introduce material from Information on STDs

HIV/STD transmission

Illegal Drugs and HIV/STD Discussion
Introduce material from Information on Alcohol and Other Drugs
Review Doorways Activity

HIV/STD prevention

Social Situations Activity
Review Talking About Condoms with Young Teens
Review Talking Risk Elimination and Risk Reduction
Review Bill of Rights and Responsibilities (Advanced)

HIV antibody testing

Purple Dye Activity
Review material from Information About HIV and AIDS

Psychosocial issues related to HIV/STDs

Decision Making Discussion

9th Grade

The life science of HIV, AIDS, and other STDs

Review material from Information About HIV and AIDS
Building Bodies Activity
Review material from Information on STDs

HIV/STD transmission

Level of Risk Activity
Review material from Information on Alcohol and Other Drugs
Review Doorways Activity

HIV/STD prevention

Risk-Taking Activity
Condom Boxes Activity
Review Talking About Condoms with Young Teens
Review Talking Risk Elimination and Risk Reduction
Review Bill of Rights and Responsibilities (Advanced)

HIV antibody testing

Review material from Information About HIV and AIDS

Psychosocial issues related to HIV/STDs

Emotional and Physical Safety Discussion

The Life Science of HIV and AIDS

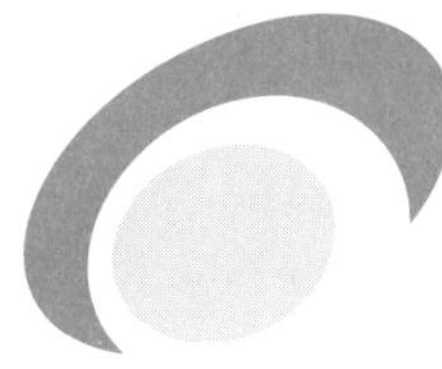

1 What is HIV?

HIV is an acronym for the name of the virus that causes AIDS.

HIV - Human Immunodeficiency Virus

H Humans, not other kinds of mammals.

I Immunodeficiency, meaning a weakening of the body's immune system. The immune system is the body's defense system against many diseases including those caused by bacteria, viruses and cancer.

V Virus, the smallest living microorganism (germ). It contains its own genetic material and must invade the body's cells in order to reproduce itself, or replicate.

2 If HIV is a virus, what is AIDS?

AIDS - Acquired Immune Deficiency Syndrome

A Acquired, meaning to get or obtain.

I Immune, referring to the immune system.

D Deficiency, meaning weakened or inadequate.

S Syndrome, refers to a group of symptoms and signs that collectively indicate the presence of a disease with various manifestations.

It is important to note that HIV and AIDS are not the same thing. AIDS refers to a clinical illness with certain signs and symptoms. HIV is the specific virus that causes that illness.

AIDS is diagnosed when an individual is infected with HIV and has one of several unusual opportunistic infections or cancers and/or has an abnormally low helper T-cell count that puts the person at risk for a life threatening illness. Helper T-cells are a specific type of white blood cell that HIV infects and kills.

According to the Centers for Disease Control and Prevention, AIDS case definition includes all HIV-infected adolescents and adults aged > 13 years who have either a) <200 CD4+ T-lymphocytes per microliter of blood (1/5000th of a teaspoon); b) a CD4+ T-lymphocyte percentage of total lymphocytes of <14%; or c) any of the identified opportunistic infections.

3 How does HIV cause AIDS?

Once HIV enters the body, the virus primarily attacks a family of white blood cells known as T-cells. There are many types of T-cells, and two important ones are helper T-cells and killer T-cells. The helper T-cells assist in regulating the immune system's functions. The killer T-cells actually destroy invading organisms that can make the body sick.

After entering the body, HIV attaches to a white blood cell, penetrates the cell, and incorporates its viral genetic material into the DNA of that white blood cell. The virus then takes control of the white blood cell's replication process. The infected cell now creates new viruses until there are too many viruses for the cell to contain and the host cell ruptures and dies. The new viruses then infect more cells, continuing the destructive cycle. This active replication process begins at the onset of HIV infection.

AIDS is diagnosed when an individual is infected with HIV and has one of several unusual opportunistic infections or cancers and/or has an abnormally low helper T-cell count that puts the person at risk for a life threatening illness.

4 How long does it take a person infected with HIV to develop signs or symptoms of AIDS?

The time period between HIV infection and developing AIDS is highly variable. Most individuals with HIV infection begin to develop mild symptoms (usually skin rashes or mouth/teeth problems but occasionally more severe symptoms like fever, weight loss, and diarrhea) between five and ten years after being infected, particularly if the person is not receiving medical treatment. However, some individuals with HIV infection develop symptoms as early as the first year, while others do not experience any symptoms for ten or more years.

Through a blood test, it is possible for medical professionals to detect the amount of virus (viral load) in people with HIV infection. The test is very good at predicting who will develop symptoms quickly and who will develop symptoms slowly. In addition, when individuals infected with HIV take specific medications, the viral load can predict who is experiencing successful responses. The process of monitoring changes in a person's viral load is currently the most accurate predictor of disease progression.

5 If a person is infected with HIV by someone who already has AIDS, will he/she develop AIDS immediately?

No. The virus (HIV) is transmissible, not AIDS. The signs and symptoms of AIDS take time to develop.

6 Do people die from AIDS?

No. People don't actually die from the HIV virus itself, or AIDS, but from a subsequent, complicating infection or illness as part of AIDS. After infection, the progression of the disease varies from person to person depending upon how rapidly that individual's immune system is destroyed by the virus.

People die from infections such as an unusual form of pneumonia caused by the organism pneumocystis carninii. These diseases are called opportunistic infections because they take advantage of the opportunity to invade the body once HIV has weakened the immune system.

7 How and where did HIV originate?

No one knows for sure where HIV came from. However, it is believed that HIV originated in Africa and was transmitted from monkeys to humans, perhaps through animal bites, scratches or consumption of animal meat. In the late-1980s, it became clear that HIV infection was an epidemic of global proportions.

8 When will there be a cure and/or a preventive vaccine for HIV?

The scientific community does not have an exact answer to this question. Many people are working very hard on developing a cure and/or a vaccine. However, the research and development for new treatments, cures and preventive vaccines is very complicated and there may not be a cure or a vaccine until well into the twenty-first century.

9 Is there any treatment for HIV and AIDS?

Yes. There are medications that can help reduce the amount of HIV replicating in the body. Anti-viral medications like reverse transcriptase inhibitors and non nucleoside reverse transcriptase inhibitors block the enzyme that helps HIV replicate. Recently a powerful and new class of medication called protease inhibitors became available. Protease inhibitors block another enzyme that is necessary for viral reproduction.

None of these medications is very effective for long when taken by themselves; however, combinations of three or more of these have been found to be extremely effective. So called "combination therapy" has led to significant, positive changes in the viral load of HIV infected people. In the majority of cases, researchers have documented the reduction of HIV in circulation to "undetectable levels" in patients who regularly take their medications. With combination therapy, some people who were close to dying have returned to good health for up to four or five years. Immune systems improve markedly with combination therapy as well. While this is very exciting, it is unlikely that HIV will be curable for most individuals in the near future. Therefore, it is still critical that people avoid getting infected in the first place.

10 Is AIDS a gay (homosexual) male disease?

No. Anyone can get HIV if his/her blood or mucous membranes directly contact the blood, semen, pre-ejaculatory fluid, vaginal secretions or breast milk of an HIV-infected person. Issues like sexual orientation, religious persuasion, race or ethnic background have to do with people, not viruses. HIV is a virus and does not discriminate against any group of individuals.

11 Is AIDS a disease that only affects people who inject illegal drugs?

No. Anyone who shares needles is at risk for HIV infection. Needles are used to inject legal and illegal drugs, vitamins, and other substances; as well as for tattooing, body piercing and other activities.

HIV Transmission

1 Which body fluids can transmit HIV?

HIV can be transmitted through the blood, semen, pre-ejaculatory fluid, vaginal secretions and/or breast milk of an infected person.

2 How does HIV transmission occur?

HIV is transmitted through contact with specific fluids, not through the air.

HIV transmission can occur in any situation in which there is contact between the infectious fluids (blood, vaginal secretions, semen, pre-ejaculatory fluid and breast milk) of an HIV-infected person and the blood and/or mucous membranes of another person.

HIV can also be transmitted from a pregnant woman to her baby during pregnancy or delivery.

3 What is a mucous membrane?

A mucous membrane is a thin lining covering certain parts of the body that are not covered by skin but which come into contact with air, such as the inside of the mouth.

The following body parts are mucous membranes that allow HIV to pass into the body. These membranes do not need to be damaged for HIV infection to occur if they are exposed to infectious fluids:

- The membrane lining the vagina, cervix and uterus
- the membrane lining the opening of the urethra at the tip of the penis
- the area underneath the foreskin of an uncircumcised penis
- the membrane lining the anus
- the membrane lining the mouth, gums and throat
- the membrane lining the inside of the nose
- the membrane lining the inside of the eyes (the pink membranes rather than the white part or the pupil)

4 Which common body fluids do not transmit HIV?

Pure tears, mucous from the nose, saliva, sweat, and urine do not transmit HIV.

5 What are some examples of behaviors that put people at risk for HIV?

The following list is a partial overview of behaviors that can put one at risk of HIV transmission:

- sexual intercourse — vaginal, anal and/or oral
- needle sharing for injection drug use, tattooing, or body piercing
- getting potentially infectious fluids into mucous membranes or cuts during first aid or trauma situations
- becoming blood brothers/blood sisters
- receiving a transfusion of infected blood or blood products (risk is now extremely low in the United States)
- being born to an HIV-infected woman
- being breast fed by an HIV-infected woman

6 Can HIV enter the body through intact skin?

No. HIV cannot pass through intact normal skin. HIV is transmitted through direct contact between the blood, vaginal secretions, semen, pre-ejaculatory fluid and/or breast milk of an HIV-infected person and another person's blood or mucous membranes.

As is the case with most infections, the skin keeps HIV out of the body. In the case of a person infected with HIV, the skin also keeps the virus inside the body.

7 How long can HIV live outside the human body?

HIV dies quite quickly outside the body, although the rate at which it dies is often dependent on environmental factors.

8 Can HIV be transmitted through a mixture of tears and blood?

Yes. Since blood can transmit HIV, it does not matter what other non-infectious fluid(s), like tears, are mixed with the blood or other infectious fluids.

9 Can you get HIV from, or give HIV to animals and/or insects?

No. HIV is the Human Immunodeficiency Virus — a human disease. Humans can neither give this virus to, nor get it from, animals like cats or dogs or insects like mosquitoes or ticks.

10 Can a person become infected with HIV by swimming in a pool used by people with AIDS?

No. Public health protocols regarding the cleanliness of pools require treatments that kill HIV.

11 Can you get HIV from tattooing or other kinds of body piercing? How about from giving blood?

It depends. There is no risk of HIV transmission so long as sterile needles and instruments are used for tattooing or body piercing. However, HIV can be transmitted if needles or instruments are reused or shared.

Likewise, giving (donating) blood is not risky because only sterile needles are used to draw blood.

12 Can you get HIV from injecting drugs

Yes. Sharing needles to inject legal or illegal drugs poses a significant risk of HIV infection.

13 Are all babies born to HIV-infected women necessarily infected with HIV at birth?

No. A baby born to an HIV-infected woman in the United States has about a one-in-four chance of being born infected with HIV. If the mother knows about her HIV infection and takes appropriate medicine during the pregnancy, the chance of perinatal transmission from mother to child drops to one-in-twelve with AZT, or even less with combination therapy.

HIV infection from mother to baby during pregnancy or birth is called perinatal transmission. Breastfeeding is another way that mother-to-child transmission occurs. Babies born to HIV-positive women have maternal antibodies to HIV in their blood. Babies who become infected with HIV will also begin to manufacture their own HIV antibodies. Babies who remain uninfected will not make antibodies to HIV and are not immune. Tests that determine the amount of HIV in the blood or identify HIV genetic material usually can tell within a few months after birth whether or not an infant is infected with HIV.

If the father is HIV-positive and the mother remains uninfected the baby will not be born with HIV.

14 What are the effects of HIV on children?

HIV affects children in somewhat different ways than adults. In particular, the virus can interfere with children's growth and development. An HIV infected child may also suffer significant neurological effects because the virus can interfere with normal brain functions. Children tend to show signs and symptoms of illness more quickly than adults do.

HIV also impacts children who become orphaned when their parents die of AIDS.

HIV Prevention

1 Can HIV be prevented?

HIV can be prevented through consistently using risk elimination or risk reduction strategies.

Risk elimination is the safest prevention choice and means that you avoid contact with potentially infectious blood, semen, pre-ejaculatory fluid, vaginal secretions and/or breast milk. This means not participating in any risky sexual activity or injection drug use. In other words, if you don't do it, you can't get HIV.

However, risk elimination is not necessarily feasible or desirable for everyone. Therefore, risk reduction (such as the use of effective barriers or sterile needles) can play an important role in HIV prevention. Unlike risk elimination, risk reduction practices cannot guarantee safety. However, latex condoms, when used consistently and correctly, can significantly reduce the chance of HIV transmission.

2 If individuals lack access to sterile needles, what can they do to decrease their risk of getting HIV when injecting?

The only 100% safe option is not to use dirty needles. In other words: stop any kind of needle sharing (including injecting drugs, tattooing or body piercing) and always use clean needles.

With regard to injection drug use, if a person is unable to discontinue injecting drugs, tattooing or body piercing, he/she should use clean needles and be sure not to share needles or other injection drug paraphernalia, such as cotton filters, cookers or water, with other users. If new needles are not available, people should only re-use their own and clean them with clean, full-strength liquid bleach.

To properly disinfect equipment, the following procedure must be followed: draw clean water through the needle into the syringe, shake 30 times, and push the water out, do this two more times; second, draw clean, full-strength liquid bleach through the needle into the syringe, shake 30 times, and push the bleach out, do this two more times; third, draw clean water through the needle into the syringe, shake 30 times, and push the water out, do this two more times.

HIV Antibody Testing

1 How can a person know if he/she is infected with HIV?

People infected with HIV are not recognizable by their appearance, physical condition and/or lifestyle. The HIV antibody test is the most commonly used test used in determining the presence of HIV infection.

2 What is the HIV antibody test?

The HIV antibody test is a blood test that identifies HIV antibodies which will be detectable in the blood of almost all HIV-infected persons three months after getting infected. However, since it takes time for the immune system to make antibodies, a test done too early, such as within twelve weeks of exposure to HIV, might not show the antibodies even though the virus was already there. It can be a good idea to get an HIV test three and six months after exposure.

There are also urine and saliva tests for HIV; however, these tests are not used as commonly as the blood test.

3 What should a person do if he/she thinks that he/she might have HIV?

The best thing to do would be to go to a health care clinic, HIV antibody testing site, or a doctor's office and talk with the medical professionals about his or her concerns. These are also places where HIV antibody testing and counseling is available. Some clinics have HIV testing and counseling protocols especially designed for youth.

One certain way to know if a person has HIV is to have an HIV antibody test. It is best to have the test done in a supportive atmosphere with compassionate professionals. However, home tests are now available.

It is important for a person to continue to protect himself or herself by practicing risk reduction or risk elimination while waiting to take the test, waiting to get test results or after receiving the results.

4 What is the difference between confidential and anonymous HIV antibody testing?

Confidential testing is the most common type of HIV antibody testing available at doctors' offices, many health clinics and hospitals. With this type of testing the person who gives the test knows the client's name, and the client's test results go into his or her medical file or a special safe according to the protocols of the test site. Therefore, the testing procedure is confidential between the health care professional and the client. The major benefit of confidential testing is that the client can have his/her test done, and results delivered, by someone with whom he/she already has a trusting and supportive relationship.

Clinics that offer anonymous testing can be located through local health departments. Anonymous test sites are less common than confidential test sites and are typically available in most urban areas. With this type of testing no one knows the client's name. The client and his/her blood are assigned a code that allows health care professionals to give the client his/her test results. These test results are not traceable back to the client's name and identity. The major benefit of anonymous testing is that no one, except the client, knows his/her test results.

In many places HIV antibody testing is offered free or at a discounted cost.

Statistics on HIV, AIDS and other STDs

- The World Health Organization estimates that 36.1 million adults and children were living with HIV infection and AIDS as of 1999.

UNAIDS/WHO, *AIDS epidemic update: December 2000*. 2000, UNAIDS/WHO: Geneva, Switzerland.

- The estimated annual incidence of curable STDs (not including AIDS and other viral STDs) is 333 million cases worldwide.

WHO Initiative on HIV/AIDS and Sexually Transmitted Infections (HSI), *Sexually Transmitted Diseases (STDs) - Fact Sheet* (April 1996).

- As of June 2000, The Centers for Disease Control and Prevention reported that 431,924 individuals are living with HIV infection and AIDS in the United States.

Centers for Disease Control and Prevention, *HIV/AIDS Surveillance Report* (2000). 12(1).

- There are an estimated 250,000 Americans who are unaware that they are HIV-infected, and many of them are young people.

Office of National AIDS Policy, *Youth and HIV/AIDS 2000: A New American Agenda* (2000).

- In the United States, half of all new HIV infections are thought to occur in young people under 25 years of age.

Office of National AIDS Policy, *Youth and HIV/AIDS 2000: A New American Agenda* (2000).

- More than 123,000 young adults in the United States have developed AIDS in their twenties. The delay between HIV infection and the onset of AIDS means that most of these young people were infected with HIV as teenagers.

Office of National AIDS Policy, *Youth and HIV/AIDS 2000: A New American Agenda* (2000).

- Although, the total number of youth in the United States who have been infected with HIV is unknown, public health officials believe that 20,000 people between 13 and 24 years of age are infected with HIV every year ñ at the rate of about 2 every hour.

Office of National AIDS Policy, *Youth and HIV/AIDS 2000: A New American Agenda* (2000).

- In the United States, more females than males are now being diagnosed with HIV in the 13-19 year old age group.

Office of National AIDS Policy, *Youth and HIV/AIDS 2000: A New American Agenda* (2000).

- By 12th grade, 65% of American youth are sexually active, and one in five has had four or more sexual partners.

Office of National AIDS Policy, *Youth and HIV/AIDS 2000: A New American Agenda* (2000).

- In the United States, 25% of high school students who have had sex said they were under the influence of alcohol and other drugs the last time they had sex.

Office of National AIDS Policy, *Youth and HIV/AIDS 2000: A New American Agenda* (2000).

- HIV infection is usually contracted sexually among American young people.

Office of National AIDS Policy, *Youth and HIV/AIDS 2000: A New American Agenda* (2000).

- The percentage of high school students who say they have had sexual intercourse decreased from 54% in 1991 to 50% in 1999. The percentage of sexually active high school students who say they used a condom the last time they had sex increased from 46% to 58% during the same period. Their accounts were confirmed when, in 1999, births to teenagers fell to their lowest rate ion 60 years.

Office of National AIDS Policy, *Youth and HIV/AIDS 2000: A New American Agenda* (2000).

continued

- About one in 50 juniors and seniors in American high schools admitted injecting illegal drugs.

Office of National AIDS Policy, *Youth and HIV/AIDS 2000: A New American Agenda* (2000).

- Each year, three million adolescents in the United States contract sexually transmitted diseases (STDs). That's about 1 in 4 sexually experienced teens. Of the 12 million Americans with STDs, about two-thirds are young people under the age of 25.

Office of National AIDS Policy, *Youth and HIV/AIDS 2000: A New American Agenda* (2000).

- Sexually transmitted diseases affect people in both developing and industrialized countries. Those aged 20-24 are at highest risk of infection. STDs have important repercussions on reproductive health and have been shown to increase the risk of infection with the AIDS virus. This is particularly serious as in many cases STDs are asymptomatic in both sexes, particularly in women.

WHO Initiative on HIV/AIDS and Sexually Transmitted Infections (HSI), *Sexually Transmitted Diseases (STDs) - Fact Sheet* (April 1996).

- Data from the 1997 Youth Risk Behavior Survey-Middle School show that:

  13% of students reported ever having had sexual intercourse (10% of sixth graders, 13% of seventh graders, and 17% of eighth graders).

  46% of sexually active students reported having had sexual intercourse with three or more partners (44% of sixth graders, 43% of seventh graders, and 46% of eighth graders).

  62% of sexually active students reported using a condom at last sexual intercourse (61% of sixth graders, 58% of seventh graders, and 66% of eighth graders).

  25% of sexually active students reported having had a sexually transmitted disease (33% of sixth graders, 23% of seventh graders, and 20% of eighth graders).

  31% of sexually active students reported drinking alcohol or using drugs before last sexual intercourse (26% of sixth graders, 38% of seventh graders, and 28% of eighth graders).

  50% of students reported ever drinking alcohol (34% of sixth graders, 55% of seventh graders, and 61% of eighth graders).

  18% of students reported ever smoking marijuana (9% of sixth graders, 19% of seventh graders, and 25% of eighth graders).

  15% of students reported sniffing glue or other inhalants (15% of sixth graders, 18% of seventh graders, and 13% of eighth graders).

J. V. Fetro, et al.,"Health-Risk Behaviors among Middle School Students in a Large Majority-Minority School District, " *Journal of School Health*, 71 (1): 30-7.

- Preventative measures have resulted in highly significant decreases in perinatal HIV transmission (HIV transmission from an infected mother to her child during pregnancy, delivery or breastfeeding) in the United States since the mid-1990s.

CDC-NCHSTP, *Status of Perinatal HIV Prevention in the U.S. Declines Continue: Hope for Extending Success to Developing World*, CDC-NCHSTP-Division of HIV/AIDS Prevention: (1998).

- Each year, between 40,000 and 80,000 Americans become infected with HIV.

Office of National AIDS Policy, *Youth & HIV/AIDS: An American Agenda, A Report to the President*. National AIDS Fund (1996).

How STDs Affect the Risk of HIV Transmission

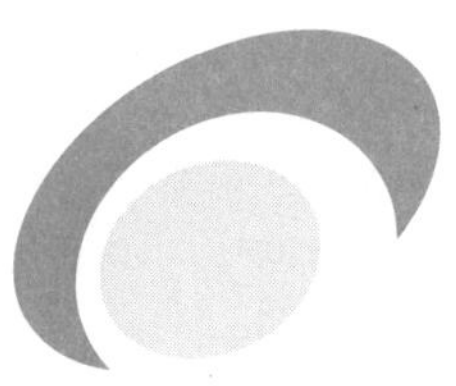

The presence of a STD in the body increases a person's chance of contracting HIV by two to five times [1]. This is especially true of any STD that produces sores or weeping lesions, such as herpes, syphilis, or chancroid. But any STD, whether it produces sores or not, will increase the risk of being exposed to HIV and may increase the risk of transmission if one, or both, of the partners are infected with HIV.

What Should a Person Do in Case of Possible Infection?

A person should visit a doctor, nurse or medical clinic as soon as possible. There are tests and treatments available for every STD, and many can be cured. Most STD tests are simple and can be done right in the doctor's office (including examinations by sight, Pap smears, cultures and blood tests). It is important that patients give doctors or nurses honest, detailed information about symptoms and/or sexual partners and it is important that partners also seek medical attention right away. STDs can be re-contracted from an untreated partner, possibly making the situation more serious.

Taking Care of Your Health

Once sexually active, it is essential for a person to take care of his/her sexual and reproductive well-being. For women, that means good hygiene and yearly pelvic and breast exams. For men, that means good hygiene and regular medical exams.

Detailed Information

Chancroid

Long-term effects

If left untreated, chancroid can cause painful and serious damage to tissue in the groin area and can lead to the formation of localized areas of infection called abscesses.

Symptoms

Painful lesions on the penis or around the opening of the vagina.

Transmission

The bacteria that cause chancroid are transmitted through unprotected sexual intercourse.

Treatment

Curable with antibiotics.

Effects on pregnant women and fetuses

If a woman has open genital sores during delivery, babies can be infected.

Increases risk of HIV transmission

Yes.

Chlamydia

Long-term effects

If left untreated for long periods of time, chlamydia in women can cause pelvic inflammatory disease (PID), damage to reproductive organs, tubal (ectopic) pregnancies and even sterility. In men, it can cause inflammation of the testicles and sterility. In both sexes, it can cause arthritis if left untreated.

Symptoms

Most women are asymptomatic. But symptoms may include increased vaginal discharge, painful urination and unusual vaginal bleeding. Symptoms in men include a burning sensation during urination and a clear-to-white urethral discharge. Men sometimes have no symptoms.

Transmission

The bacteria that cause chlamydia are transmitted through unprotected sexual contact with the penis, vagina, anus or mouth.

Effects on pregnant women and fetuses

Chlamydia can cause tubal (ectopic) pregnancies and can infect babies during birth, causing eye infections or pneumonia.

Treatment

Curable with antibiotics.

Increases risk of HIV transmission

Yes.

Genital Herpes

Long-term effects

The herpes virus stays in the body for life and may cause repeated outbreaks of sores. In rare cases, it can lead to blindness if it is brought to the eyes, usually by a hand that has touched an infected area.

Symptoms

Painful sores in the penile, vaginal, anal or oral areas. Sores can also be on the cervix or inside the urethra. Sores generally break open, scab, and heal within a period of weeks or days.

Transmission

The virus that causes genital herpes is transmitted through unprotected sexual contact with the penis, vagina, anus or mouth. Open sores make transmission more likely but do not need to be present for transmission to occur.

Treatment

No cure is available for herpes. The drug Acyclovir and others can significantly reduce outbreaks, lessening their frequency, duration and severity.

Effects on pregnant women and fetuses

If a woman has open sores during delivery, herpes cam infect babies and can cause blindness or damage to their central nervous system.

Increases risk of HIV transmission

Yes.

Genital Warts

Long-term effects

The virus that causes genital warts (Human Papilloma Virus-HPV) can stay with the body for life, even after the removal of warts. The virus has been associated with an increased risk of cancer of the cervix, vulva, penis and anus.

Symptoms

Small painless hard spots or bumps inside or outside of the vagina, on the cervix or penis or around the anus. Sometimes there are no symptoms.

Transmission

The virus that causes genital warts is transmitted through unprotected sexual or other contact with the warts.

Treatment

The warts can be removed with caustic ointments or surgery but the virus HPV can remain in the body for life.

Effects on pregnant women and growing fetuses

Babies can get infected in their throats or genitals during birth.

Increases risk of HIV transmission

No.

Gonorrhea

Long-term effects

In women, if left untreated for long periods of time, gonorrhea can lead to painful infection of the pelvic area (PID), arthritis, tubal (ectopic) pregnancies and even sterility. In men, it can lead to discharge, burning during urination, chronic prostate infection and arthritis. If brought to the eyes, usually by a hand that has touched an infected area, it can lead to blindness.

Symptoms

Many women are asymptomatic, have mild symptoms or confuse them with other conditions. As the disease progresses in women, there may be a burning sensation during urination or abdominal pain. Infections in the throat can cause swollen glands. Many men will have a white, yellowish or greenish discharge from the penis and burning during urination.

Transmission

The bacteria that cause gonorrhea are transmitted through unprotected sexual contact with the penis, vagina, anus or mouth and are highly contagious.

Treatment

Curable with antibiotics.

Effects on pregnant women and fetuses

Women with gonorrhea are more likely to give birth prematurely. During birth, gonorrhea can infect the eyes of babies and can eventually cause blindness.

Increases risk of HIV transmission

Yes.

Granuloma Inguinale (GI)

Long-term effects

If left untreated, GI lesions can spread to cover the entire pubic area. The lesions can bleed and lead to secondary infections that can be highly damaging.

Symptoms

Painless lesions on the vulva and vagina in women, and painless lesions on the penis, scrotum and groin in men.

Transmission

The bacteria that cause GI are transmitted through unprotected sexual contact.

Treatment

Curable with antibiotics.

Effects on pregnant women and fetuses

Uncertain.

Increases risk of HIV transmission

Yes.

Hepatitis B

Long-term effects

Most people heal completely, but serious complications, such as chronic hepatitis, cirrhosis or cancer of the liver, or death may occur.

Symptoms

Over half of infected people have no symptoms. But symptoms include yellowing of the skin, nausea, cramps and extreme tiredness. Some people experience intense flu-like symptoms.

Transmission

Like HIV, the virus that causes hepatitis B is transmitted through unprotected sexual contact as well as needle sharing.

Treatment

Treatment is available; however, some people do not respond to it.

Effects on pregnant women and fetuses

Babies may become infected during birth and become life-long carriers of hepatitis B, or they may contract a full-blown, life-threatening case of the disease.

Increases risk of HIV transmission

No.

Pelvic Inflammatory Disease (PID): (Only Affects Women)

Long-term effects

If left untreated, PID can cause damage to the fallopian tubes, which can lead to sterility, tubal (ectopic) pregnancies and, in some cases, potentially fatal inflammation of the abdominal cavity.

Symptoms

Abdominal pain, fever, increased vaginal discharge and menstrual flow, vomiting, tiredness.

Transmission

The bacteria that cause PID are transmitted through unprotected sexual intercourse. PID can also develop as a result of other untreated STDs.

Treatment

Curable with antibiotics.

Effects on pregnant women and fetuses

PID can cause tubal (ectopic) pregnancies and sterility.

Increases risk of HIV transmission

Yes.

Pubic Lice (Crabs) and Scabies

Long-term effects

Discomfort and infection of others.

Symptoms

Intense itching in genital area and/or anywhere there is body hair.

Transmission

Pubic lice and scabies are parasites transmitted through sexual or other contact with an infected person or his/her personal effects such as bed sheets, underclothing or towels.

Treatment

Curable with over-the-counter shampoos and creams.

Effects on pregnant women and growing fetuses

None.

Increases risk of HIV transmission

No.

Syphilis

Long-term effects

Left untreated for many years, syphilis can cause blindness, heart disease, spinal cord damage, chronic dementia, and, eventually, death.

Symptoms

There are three stages to syphilis. The first stage, which lasts only a week or two, involves a painless sore (chancre) in the area of the penis, vagina, anus or mouth. After the sore heals, the disease enters the second stage where symptoms include rashes, fever, swollen joints and hair loss. This also lasts only a week or two. In the third phase, there are no symptoms, but after 30 years or more, severe organ damage occurs that can affect almost any organ system including the heart, liver and brain.

Transmission

The bacteria that cause syphilis are transmitted through unprotected sexual contact.

Treatment

Curable with antibiotics.

Effects on pregnant women and fetuses

Fetuses can become infected with syphilis. This may cause miscarriage, stillbirth, mental retardation or many physical deformities.

Increases risk of HIV transmission

Yes.

Trichomoniasis

Long-term effects

Left untreated, trichomoniasis can cause abnormal pap smears, chronic vaginal irritation and pain during intercourse.

Symptoms

Women generally have a thick, frothy, foul-smelling vaginal discharge. Men generally do not have any symptoms, but may have some inflammation and/or milky penile discharge.

Transmission

The parasites that cause trichomoniasis are transmitted through unprotected sexual contact with the penis, vagina, anus or mouth. The parasites can also be transmitted through contact with toilet seats, wet towels and clothing.

Treatment

Curable with antibiotics.

Effects on pregnant women and fetuses

None.

Increases risk of HIV transmission

Yes.

HIV/STD Transmission and Alcohol and Other Drugs

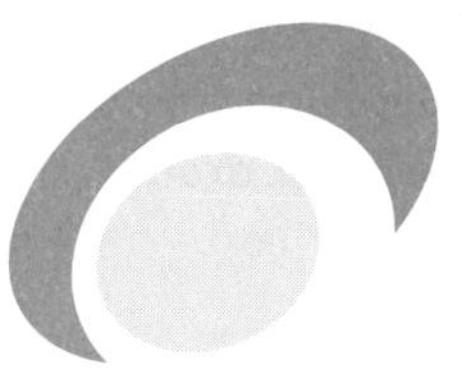

The use of alcohol and other drugs can directly and indirectly increase one's risk of HIV/STD infection and pregnancy.

Direct transmission of HIV can occur when there is contact between one person's infectious bodily fluids (blood, vaginal secretions, semen, pre-ejaculatory fluid, and breast milk) and another person's blood or mucous membranes. Needle sharing during injection drug use puts a person at risk of direct HIV transmission.

Indirect transmission of HIV can occur when there is mediated contact between one person's infectious bodily fluids (blood, vaginal secretions, semen, pre-ejaculatory fluid and breast milk) and another person's blood or mucous membranes, such as through sharing water or cotton filters while injecting drugs. Using alcohol and other drugs can indirectly increase the risk of HIV/STD infection by facilitating unsafe behaviors such as unprotected sex or physical violence.

While alcohol is legal for adults over the age of 21, all the other drugs listed in this appendix are illegal for everyone. Using them can have serious legal as well as health consequences.

Detailed Information

Alcohol

Effects on the body

Alcohol is a depressant, which means it slows down body functions. It also slows down thought processes and reaction time, making driving under the influence of alcohol extremely dangerous. Excess drinking can lead to vomiting and unconsciousness. Long-term abuse can lead to damage of the liver, heart or brain.

Effects in behavior

Alcohol often makes people feel less inhibited, more daring and "invincible." It can lead to unintended sexual activity and/or violent behavior. Alcohol can also impair judgement because of confusion.

Increased risk of disease transmission

Directly: No. There is no risk of transmitting HIV or STDs by sharing drinks or glasses.

Indirectly: Yes. Drinking alcohol can lead to risky behavior such as increased sexual activity, unprotected sex, and violence. These behaviors increase the risk of HIV/STD infection.

Amphetamines

Effects on the body

Amphetamines are stimulants. They give people energy and sometimes reduce appetite. Long-term abuse can lead to sleeplessness, loss of appetite and sometimes collapse.

Effects on behavior

Amphetamines bring users "up," making them wide-awake and alert. Amphetamines are often used along with other drugs, allowing the user to stay awake and aware to experience fully the effects of those other drugs. Amphetamines are highly addictive.

Increased risk of disease transmission

Directly: Yes. Injecting amphetamines can lead to increased risk of direct transmission of HIV and other blood-borne STDs through sharing needles, syringes or other drug injection paraphernalia.

Indirectly: Yes. Taking amphetamine pills or powder along with cocaine or heroin can amplify the effects of those drugs and lead to risky behaviors such as unprotected sex and violence. These behaviors increase the risk of HIV/STD transmission.

Cocaine/Crack

Effects on the body

Cocaine is a stimulant. The high lasts only 15 to 30 minutes, and afterwards, users feel tired and down. Cocaine releases "pleasure chemicals" in the brain, making users feel happy, energized and strong. Crack is a smokable form of cocaine that gives a faster, more intense yet shorter-lasting high. Long-term abuse of cocaine leads to sleeplessness, anxiety, and depression. Also, because it is highly addictive, users often find themselves financially and psychologically enslaved by the drug. Risk of overdosing is high.

Effects on behavior

The rush associated with cocaine makes people feel passionate and powerful. Some also say that it makes them feel "sexy." But the "down" that follows the rush makes people feel miserable and can make them desperate to obtain more of the drug. Use of cocaine can impair judgment because of the "sexy" feeling during the high or because of the overwhelming craving for another dose during the down. With crack, it is common for users to exchange sex for more drugs or money.

Increased risk of disease transmission

Directly: Yes. Injecting cocaine can lead to increased risk of direct transmission of HIV and other blood-borne STDs through sharing needles, syringes or other drug injection paraphernalia.

Indirectly: Yes. Snorting or smoking cocaine can lead to behaviors such as unprotected sex and violence which themselves pose a direct risk of HIV/STD infection.

Ecstacy

Effects on the Body

Ecstasy is a combination of stimulant and hallucinogen. It gives the user energy and alters his/her mental state. Severe abuse can lead to unpleasant physical and/or mental effects.

Effects on Behavior

Users feel energized and uninhibited, often sexually. Many people report feelings of warmth and affection toward other people. Use of ecstasy can impair good judgment because of the artificially strong feelings of affection and feeling that "everything's okay."

Increased risk of disease transmission

Directly: Yes. Injecting ecstacy can lead to increased risk of direct transmission of HIV and other blood-borne STDs through sharing needles, syringes or other drug injection paraphernalia.

Indirectly: Yes. Taking ecstasy in pill or powder form can lead to increased sexual activity and unprotected sex. These behaviors increase the risks of HIV/STD infection.

Heroin

Effects on the Body

Heroin is a narcotic. It makes users feel drowsy, reduces the ability to feel pain, and clouds the mind. Later, users feel sweaty and nauseated. Heroin is highly addictive.

Effects on Behavior

Heroin makes people feel relaxed and gives them an overall sense of well-being. Use of heroin can impair good judgment because of the drug-induced feeling that "everything's okay" or because of the strong craving for more heroin when the drug's effects have worn off. Risk of overdosing is high.

Increased risk of disease transmission

Directly: Yes. Injecting heroin can lead to increased risk of direct transmission of HIV and other blood-borne STDs through sharing needles, syringes or other drug injection paraphernalia.

Indirectly: Yes. Snorting or smoking heroin can impair a person's ability to practice HIV/STD prevention behavior.

LSD

Effects on the body

LSD is part stimulant and part hallucinogen. The drug increases the user's heart rate and brain activity, causing hallucinations that can last as long as twelve hours. Long-term abuse has been reported to lead to unexpected "flashbacks" for years.

Effects on behavior

LSD puts people in an altered mental state. They often see and hear things that do not exist at all. The "unreal" effects of LSD prohibit users from being able to make reasoned, informed decisions about their behavior.

Increased risk of disease transmission

Directly: No. There is no risk of transmitting HIV through ingesting LSD.

Indirectly: Yes. Ingesting LSD can lead to risky behaviors such as unprotected sex and violence. These behaviors increase the risk HIV/STD transmission.

Marijuana (and Hashish)

Effects on the body

Marijuana is a hallucinogen. However, it affects people very differently — some feel calm, some feel energized, some fall asleep, some get nervous, anxious or paranoid. Physical coordination and reaction time can be impaired. Driving under the influence of marijuana is highly dangerous. Long-term abuse can lead to lack of motivation and memory loss.

Effects on behavior

Smoking or eating marijuana alters one's mental state making people often feel that their actions do not have "real world" consequences. Use of marijuana can impair judgment because of confusion or lack of concern about consequences.

Increased risk of disease transmission

Directly: No. There is no risk of transmitting HIV or STDs by sharing pipes, bongs or joints (rolled marijuana cigarettes).

Indirectly: Yes. Smoking or eating marijuana can lead to risky behaviors such as unprotected sex, which increase the risk of HIV/STD infection.

PCP

Effects on the body

PCP is a hallucinogen. However, it may affect people as a depressant, stimulant or hallucinogen. PCP increases heart rate and respiration and decreases sensitivity to pain. Users feel dizzy and distorted and, in cases of higher dosage, can become extremely confused, agitated and violent. Long-term abuse can lead to brain damage.

Effects on Behavior

PCP can cause users to become extremely violent. Decreased sensitivity to pain can lead to injury of the user or others. Use of PCP can impair judgment because of extreme confusion or disorientation.

Increased risk of pregnancy and disease transmission

Directly: Yes. Injecting PCP can lead to increased risk of direct transmission of HIV and other blood-borne STDs through sharing needles, syringes or other drug injection paraphernalia.

Indirectly: Yes. Snorting, smoking or ingesting PCP can lead to violent behavior that results in bleeding and increased risk of exposure to HIV and other blood-borne STDs.

Steroids

Effects on the body

Steroids are hormones that control the body's metabolism. Athletes often use anabolic steroids (steroids that help to build up body tissue) to increase muscle mass. Anabolic steroids help the body metabolize food into muscle tissue; they also can weaken the immune system and, in extreme cases, lead to death.

Effects on behavior

Steroids disrupt the body's natural hormonal balance. This can lead to depression, mania and/or violence. Use of steroids can impair judgment because of the difficulty people have in handling the effects of unnatural hormone levels.

Increased risk of disease transmission

Directly: Yes. Injecting steroids can lead to increased risk of direct transmission of HIV and other blood-borne STDs through sharing needles, syringes or other drug injection paraphernalia.

Indirectly: Yes. Ingesting steroids can lead to violent behavior that results in bleeding and increased risk of HIV and other blood-borne STDs.

Activities List

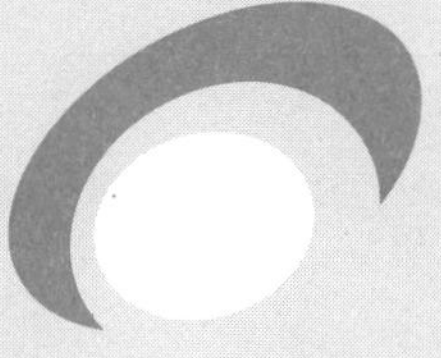

Guiding Questions

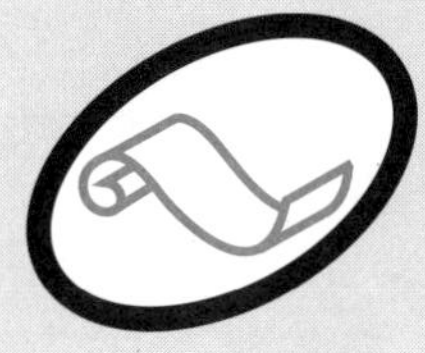

What does it mean to be responsible and respectful about students' physical and emotional health?

How do the terms health, respect, responsibility, and rights apply to students' school and home relationships?

How do the terms health, respect, responsibility, and rights apply to people's behavior with regard to HIV/STD prevention?

To whom can youth go for support or to discuss concerns regarding health?

Content: Attitudes, Skills

Recommended Grade Level: 5-9

Correlation to Standards: Health Education: 1, 4, 5, 6, 7; Science Education: F

Estimated Time: 15 minutes excluding Lesson Extension & Assessment

Materials: Basic Bill; Advanced Bill.

Part 1: The Basic Bill & the Advanced Bill

1. Use either the Basic Bill or the Advanced Bill according to your students' grade level, behaviors, developmental maturity and community norms.
2. Distribute the appropriate Bill handout to each student and/or display the Bill transparency on an overhead projector.
3. Read, or invite a student to read the Bill to the class:

(see next page for the Basic Bill and Advanced Bill)

Basic Bill for Students

- Your body is yours to respect and protect.
- You can prevent the spreading HIV and other STDs.
- You have a right to be safe from these diseases and stay healthy.
- You have the right to say "no" to anything that is not safe for you.
- For example, you have the right to say "no" to sex, or other risky behaviors such as physical fighting and using alcohol or other drugs.
- Each person has the right to say "no" to a risky activity.
- You also have the responsibility to protect other people. This means that it is not OK to put someone else in danger. It is important to respect other people's right to say "no" to you even if you feel safe.
- Sometimes people are forced to do things that they don't want to do and that are dangerous. It is not your fault if someone makes you do something that does not feel safe to you. If something unsafe happens, you always have the right to talk about it, be respected and get help. Find an adult you can trust and tell him/her what happened.
- You are a valuable person and an important part of your community.
- You deserve to be treated with respect.
- You have the right and the responsibility to protect yourself and other people against these diseases.

Advanced Bill for Students

- Your body is yours to respect and protect.
- You can prevent HIV and other STDs.
- You have the right to be safe from these diseases and stay healthy.
- You have the right to say "no" to anything that is not safe for you.

  For example, you have the right to say no to sex, or other risky behaviors such as physical fighting or using alcohol or other drugs. You don't have to do anything with your body that doesn't feel safe to you, no matter whom you're with, whether you've done it before, or what you agreed to earlier. If you choose to say "no" you don't need to justify yourself; it doesn't have to be "I don't want to because..." "I don't want to!" is enough.

- You also have the responsibility to protect other people. This means that it is not OK to put someone else in danger. You have the responsibility to communicate about whatever risks might exist. It is important to respect other people's right to say "no" to you even if you feel safe.
- If you choose to take risks, make your behavior as safe as possible — emotionally and physically.

  Emotional safety can exist when both people make the decision to engage in a certain behavior together and can say no if they want to. If you feel as if you couldn't say "no" or that your "no" wouldn't be respected, then you're not in an emotionally safe situation. The use of alcohol and other drugs can seriously affect a person's ability to make emotionally and physically safe decisions.

  Physical safety is also based on trust, respect, and communication. In terms of sexual risks, the safest choice you can make is to wait to have sex until you are in a risk-free relationship.

  Safe sex can exist, but only in a risk-free, faithful relationship where both partners get tested, know they don't have HIV or other STDs, and have no other risky behaviors.

However, if you choose to have sex before you're in a risk-free relationship, you should know that you are taking a risk. You need to protect yourself and your partner by using barriers, such as condoms. Using barriers during sex is called safer sex. Safer sex is not "safe" because the barriers do not provide 100% protection.

- Physical safety is also important in other risky situations such as needle sharing for injecting drugs, body piercing or tattooing. From a health perspective, the safest choice is not to use drugs at all and never to share needles.
- You are a valuable person and an important part of your community.
- Sometimes people are forced to do things that are dangerous. It is not your fault that someone makes you do something that does not feel safe to you. If something unsafe happens, you always have the right to talk about it, be respected and get help. Find an adult you can trust and tell him/her what happened.
- You deserve to be treated with respect.
- You have the right and the responsibility to protect yourself and other people against HIV and other STDs.

Part 2: Class Discussion

1 What are the main concepts communicated in the Bill?

2 Do students agree or disagree with these messages?

3 Do students think that they can adopt the Bill's messages? Why or why not?

4 Are there some situations where the Bill's messages might be more difficult to act upon? Why?

5 What is the meaning of the statement, "If something unsafe happens, you always have the right to talk about it, be respected and get help?"

6 To whom can students go for support?

Lesson Extension & Assessment:

1 Students develop their own Personalized Bill and present their ideas as a language arts project and/or visual art project.

2 In small groups, students develop answers for the following grammar questions without the aid of a dictionary: "What is health (noun)? What are rights (noun)? What is responsibility (noun)? What is respect (noun and verb)?" Groups discuss examples of the connections between the terms: **health, rights, responsibility,** and **respect** as they apply to one, or more, of the following words: friendship, neighborhood, family, and school. Each group creates a poster displaying examples of these connections.

3 Students write a short essay or journal entry addressing the concepts of rights and responsibilities in the context of the United Sates Constitution and Bill of Rights, the Civil Rights Movement, or the principle of Human Rights.

4 In small groups, students discuss aspects of their general safety addressing the questions listed below. Each group creates a resource list to provide accurate and appropriate referral information for local youth their age.

- What rights do youths have that protect them from physical harm?
- What rights do youths have that protect them from emotional harm?
- What can the school do to assist youths in staying safe and healthy?
- To whom can youths turn for support or to discuss concerns regarding dangerous situations?

5 In small groups, students brainstorm and make posters that display examples of real life situations where youths their age could apply the Bill's messages. Students should identify situations in which older youths could apply the Bill's messages. Also, students should identify situations in which adults could apply the Bill's messages. Display the posters.

6 In small groups students develop, practice and present a skit about a situation in which the characters' behavior demonstrates messages in the Bill. Groups perform their skits for the class and/or families and community. After the presentations, discuss the skits as a class.

7 In small groups, students outline role plays in which the characters' behavior demonstrates messages in the Bill. Groups swap outlines for role play situations. Each group develops, practices and presents a new role play based on the outline just received from another group. After the presentations, discuss the skits as a class.

8 In small groups, students write and present/record a 30 second Public Service Announcement (PSA). The PSAs should incorporate themes drawn from students' Personalized Bills.

9 Students keep their Personalized Bills in their portfolios. Students write a second Personalized Bill later in the school year. Students compare the two Bills to gain insight about personal growth.

Guiding Questions

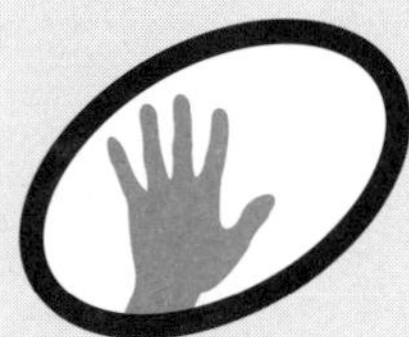

What is the relationship between female and male reproductive anatomy and physiology, human reproduction and disease transmission?

What are differences and similarities between disease prevention and pregnancy prevention?

Why is HIV/STD prevention important?

Content: Knowledge

Recommended Grade Level: 8-9

Correlation to Standards: Health Education: 1, 4, 5, 7; Science Education: A, C, F, G

Estimated Time: 25 minutes excluding Lesson Extension & Assessment

Materials: 1 condom (optional)

Part 1: HIV/STD Infection and Prevention

1. Use the following motions to present a model of the female reproductive system, the penis, the anus and the mouth.

2. Demonstrate the female reproductive system using the following progression:

    Ovaries: Make your hands into fists and hold your arms above your head in a "V" shape. Open and close a fist to represent ovulation.

    Fallopian Tubes: Start with the ovaries position. Keep your elbows stationary and lower your forearms so that your hands are touching at eye level and your forearms are parallel to the ground. As your hands move into this position they draw the path of the fallopian tubes from the ovaries to the uterus.

    Uterus: Bring the palms of your hands together. Drop your elbows down so that they are in front of your stomach, then separate the fingers and upper palm to form an open U-shape. Your elbows should be approximately three inches apart. The hands represent the sides of the uterus.

    Cervix: Without changing position, identify the cervix as the opening of the uterus, illustrated by the place where the bases of the palms touch

    Vagina: Without changing position, identify the area between the forearms as the vagina.

Vaginal Opening: Without changing position, identify the space between the elbows as the vaginal opening.

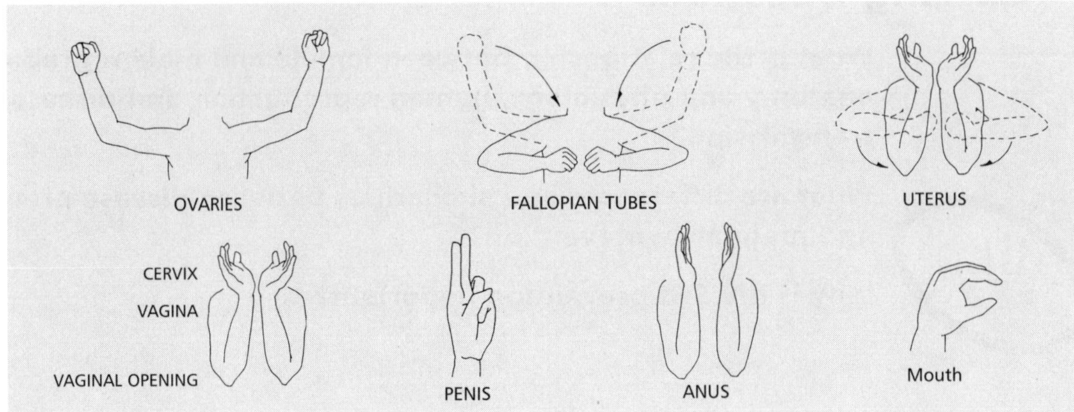

3 Demonstrate the penis by extending the index and middle fingers of one hand and keeping all of your other fingers in a fist. Illustrate the opening at the end of the penis by pointing to the space between the tips of the outstretched fingers.

4 Demonstrate the anus by holding your hands and forearms parallel, three inches apart, palms face to face, fingers pointing upward.

5 Demonstrate the mouth by making a "C" shape with your hand.

6 Review the functions of the body parts listed above:

- Ovaries - produce eggs and female hormones.
- Fallopian Tubes - connect the ovaries and the uterus; allow eggs to travel to the uterus.
- Uterus - the place where the fetus grows.
- Cervix - the base of the uterus, where the uterus opens into the vagina.
- Vagina - the birth canal, connects the uterus to the outside of the body.
- Penis - male organ for sex and urination.
- Anus - opening to the rectum.

7 Use the hand positions outlined above to describe and demonstrate the mechanisms of vaginal intercourse, anal intercourse and oral sex. Discuss the following questions and responses considering each type of intercourse:

Vaginal Intercourse:

1 Who is at risk for HIV and other STDs? Why?

Both the man and the woman are at risk. In this situation, both the penis and the vagina are vulnerable to HIV and other STDs, and can produce sexual fluids that can transmit HIV and/or have the potential to transmit other STDs on contact.

2 Who is at greater risk? Why?

In general, the woman is at greater risk than her male partner for the following reasons: There is greater surface area on the mucous membranes of the vagina than at the tip of a man's penis.

- It is more likely that there will be tearing of the vaginal membranes than of the penis during vaginal intercourse.
- After ejaculation, the man's semen typically stays inside the woman for longer than her sexual fluids are in direct contact with his penis.

3 When does the risk for STDs begin?

The risk begins on contact and increases with penetration and ejaculation.

Oral Sex:

1 Who is at risk for HIV and other STDs? Why?

Both people are at risk. In this situation, the mouth is vulnerable to HIV and other STDs when it comes into contact with the microorganisms that cause STDs and/or the sexual fluids that transmit HIV and other STDs.

2 Who is at greater risk? Why?

In general, the mouth is at greater risk than the penis, vagina or anus. The mucous membranes in the mouth are vulnerable to HIV in the sexual fluids, whereas the saliva (unless mixed with blood) does not transmit HIV. Some other STDs can be transmitted through saliva, but the risk is still higher for the mouth.

3 When does the risk for STDs begin?

The risk begins on contact and increases with penetration and ejaculation.

Anal Intercourse:

1 Who is at risk for STDs? Why?

Both partners are at risk. The person with the penis is at risk for reasons described above; the other person is at risk because the anus, like the vagina, is vulnerable to HIV and other STDs. The tissues of the anus are mucous membranes.

2 Who is at greater risk? Why?

The person with the anus is at greater risk: the anal membranes are more likely to tear, there is greater surface area compared to the opening at the tip of the penis; and the pre-ejaculatory fluid and semen are likely to remain inside the anus longer than blood or feces on the penis.

3 When does the risk for STDs begin?

The risk begins on contact and increases with penetration and ejaculation.

4. Discuss and demonstrate the location of other STDs. For example, point to the cervix, vagina, penis and anus and discuss genital warts. See Information on STDs.

5. Discuss and demonstrate disease risk reduction techniques, including the use of condoms. If age-appropriate, unroll a condom over a finger penis to show the purpose of barriers.

Part 2: Pregnancy and Prevention

1. Chart the movement and development of the fetus from conception to birth.

2. Discuss and demonstrate how, and where, birth control methods work to prevent pregnancy. For example, point to the ovaries and discuss the birth control pill. Address condoms, diaphragms, cervical caps, spermicides, IUDs, birth control pills, rhythm method, withdrawal, implants and abstinence. Note which methods provide protection against diseases (abstinence and condoms).

3. Compare and contrast disease prevention with pregnancy prevention. Discuss the role of risk elimination and risk reduction in the prevention of disease transmission and pregnancy.

4. Discuss the relative risk associated with being the penetrating partner and the receptive partner. Also, discuss the relative risk of intercourse involving penetration by a finger vs. oral sex vs. vaginal or anal intercourse.

5. Focus on the importance of disease prevention including a discussion of risk elimination and risk reduction.

Lesson Extension & Assessment

1. Working in small groups, students address social issues related to disease prevention and contraception. Which are more socially acceptable? Why? Which have more options? Why? What are some of the social factors that can make it easier or harder for people to prevent HIV/STDs and/or pregnancy? Groups organize their main points and present five minute oral summations to the class.

2. Working individually, students write journal entries about their personal responses to the public health need for disease and pregnancy prevention. Is prevention complicated or is it easy? Why? Is prevention scary? How can students transform their concerns about HIV/STD infection and/or pregnancy into motivation for prevention?

Guiding Questions

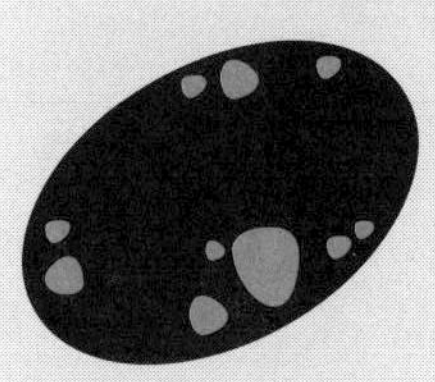

What are cells, bacteria and viruses?

How are viruses and bacteria similar? How are they different?

Why is it hard to develop a cure for HIV?

Why is it important to prevent HIV?

Content: Attitudes, Knowledge

Recommended Grade Level: 5-6

Correlation to Standards: Health Education: 1; Science Education: A, C, E, F, G

Estimated Time: 25 minutes excluding Lesson Extension & Assessment

---

Part 1: Cells, Bacteria & Antibiotic Medicine

1 What is a cell?

A cell is the basic structural unit of all living organisms.

2 What kinds of organisms have cells?

All living organisms have cells.

3 Are there different kinds of human cells?

Yes, for example there are white blood cells, red blood cells and the cells that form the skin and internal organs.

4 What are white blood cells?

White blood cells are part of the immune system and help the body fight off infections.

5 What do human cells look like?

Human cells can be different shapes, but typically they are round.

6 What are bacteria?

Bacteria are one-celled organisms that can reproduce on their own. Some bacteria cause diseases in humans.

7 What is a virus?

A virus is a very tiny organism that needs to be inside a living host cell in order to replicate. Some viruses cause diseases in humans.

8 What is an antibiotic medicine?

An antibiotic medicine is a substance that can kill, slow or prevent the growth of bacteria and other organisms that cause infectious diseases.

9 The activity space in the classroom represents a human body.

10 Three volunteers represent bacteria. Bacteria wait by the classroom door pretending to be outside the body.

11 The rest of the class divides into groups of three or four students that represent white blood cells. Students in each group face inward and link hands to form circles representing living cells; a broken circle is a dead white blood cell. White blood cells can move slowly in the body.

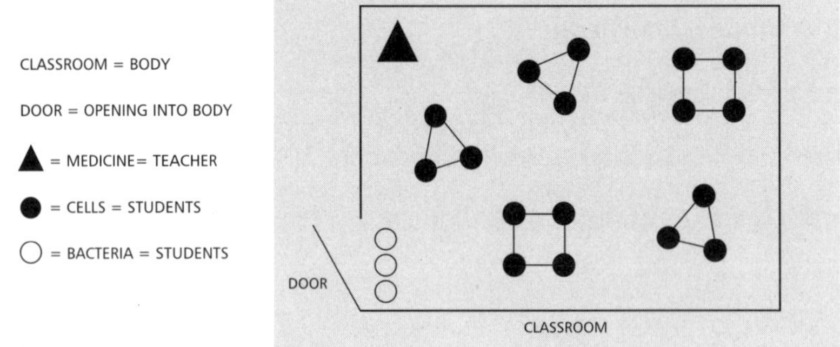

12 Bacteria enter the body and move among the white blood cells pretending to scare or attack the white blood cells for a minute or two. Bacteria can not enter white blood cells.

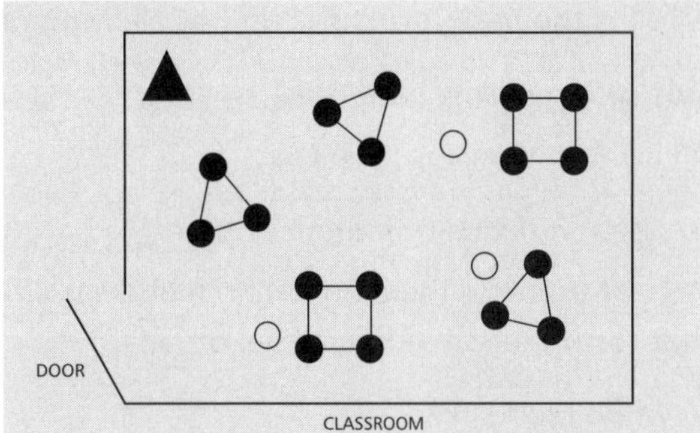

13 The teacher represents an antibiotic medicine that can kill bacteria without harming cells. The antibiotic medicine chases and tags the bacteria.

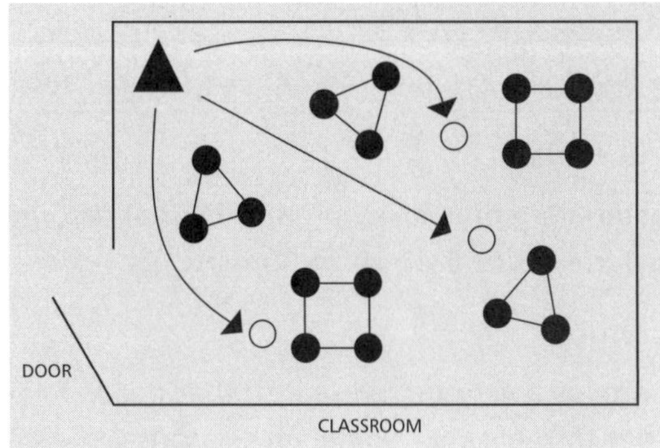

14 Once tagged, the bacteria sit on the floor and pretend to die.

15 What can antibiotic medicines do?

They can kill bacteria without harming white blood cells.

16 How can antibiotic medicines kill bacteria without harming the white blood cells?

Bacteria and white blood cells have very different functions and sensitivities. Antibiotic medicines recognize and attack bacteria, but do not hurt healthy white blood cells.

17 Has anyone (in the class) taken any antibiotic medicines? Why? Did the antibiotic medicine work?

Most likely, a student will report taking an antibiotic, recovering from the infection, and having no problems from taking the medicine itself.

18 Why is it important to complete the full course of antibiotic medicine as prescribed?

The correct dose of antibiotics lasts long enough to kill all of the bacteria that cause a specific infection. If you stop taking the antibiotic medicine too soon, those bacteria that are still alive sometimes cause a second wave of infection that might be resistant to the antibiotic taken earlier. This situation can be dangerous for the person with the infection as well as for other people who get infected with the resistant bacteria which are harder to kill.

Part 2: White Blood Cells and HIV

1 What is HIV?

HIV is the Human Immunodeficiency Virus, an identifiable virus that weakens the immune systems of humans.

2 What kind of cells does HIV usually infect?

HIV infects white blood cells that are an important part of the immune system.

3 The students who were bacteria now represent HIV. As in Part 1, they stand by the doorway to the human body (the classroom).

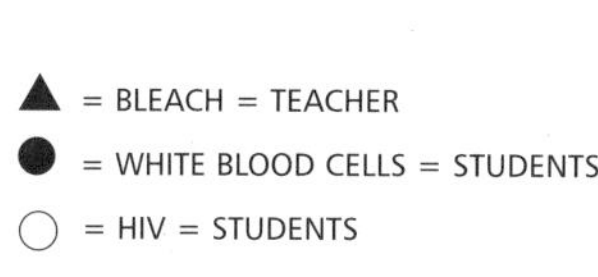

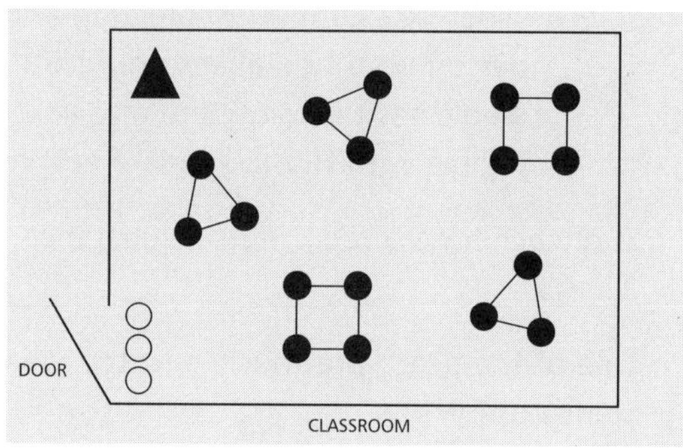

4 HIV moves among the white blood cells. Each HIV can enter one white blood cell. White blood cells cannot keep HIV out. Once HIV is in a white blood cell, the virus cannot leave to infect another white blood cell. At least two white blood cells remain uninfected.

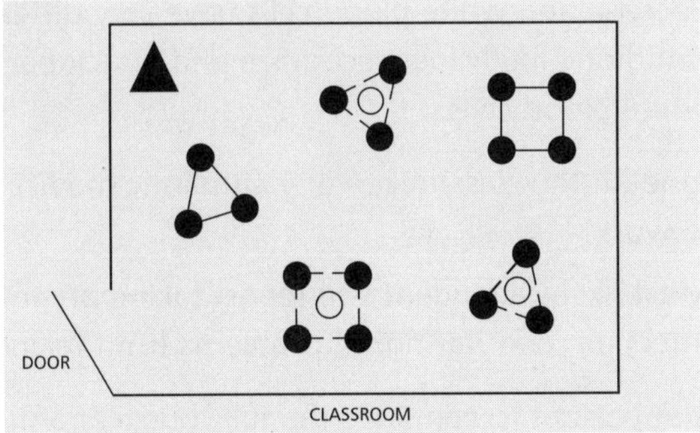

5 Infected white blood cells demonstrate how HIV kills them by sitting down on the floor. HIV inside these white blood cells remain standing.

6 Now, one HIV from a dead white blood cell selects and infects a healthy white blood cell. One healthy white blood cell still remains uninfected.

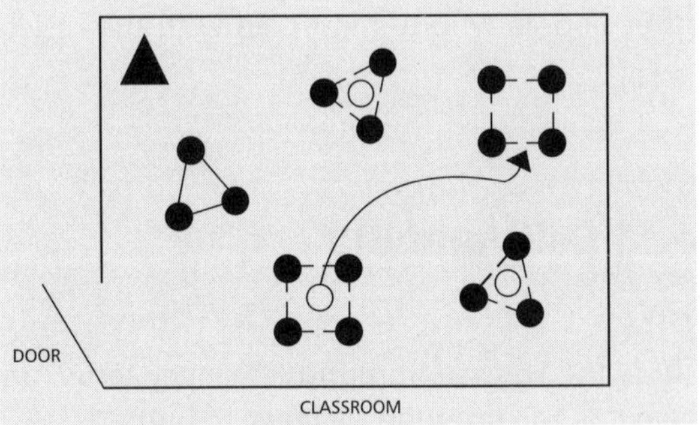

7 The newly infected white blood cell dies. The HIV remains standing. The healthy white blood cell is still standing.

8 What does HIV do to white blood cells?

It kills them.

9 What happens when HIV kills a person's white blood cells?

When HIV continues infecting and killing a person's white blood cells, the person won't be able to fight off other infections and may die. Special medicines that slow the rate at which HIV kills white blood cells can help people with HIV live longer and healthier.

10 The teacher now represents a substance such as bleach that is strong enough to kill HIV.

11 One of the dead, previously infected white blood cells comes back to life and stands up.

12 Bleach stands between the (now) living but infected cell and a healthy cell.

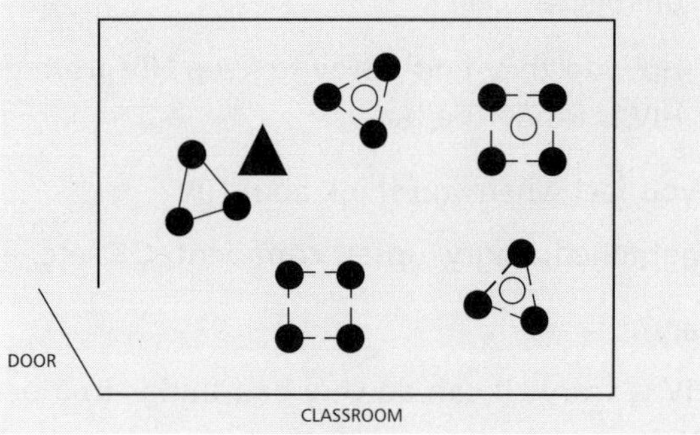

13 Bleach opens the HIV infected cell and tags the HIV.

14 The cell and HIV die.

15 Then, bleach tags the healthy cell.

16 That cell dies.

17 How can the bleach kill the HIV?

The bleach has to kill the infected cell in order to kill the HIV.

18 If bleach can kill an HIV infected cell, what will the bleach do to a nearby healthy cell?

The bleach will also kill the healthy cell.

Part 3: Wrap Up

1 What are some of the differences between bacteria and viruses?

- Bacteria are living microorganisms that can reproduce on their own; viruses need to be inside a host cell to replicate.
- Bacteria attack cells from the outside; viruses invade cells and go inside.
- Antibiotic medicine can kill bacteria inside the human body; there are no medicines that can effectively kill viruses like HIV inside a person without harming that person's cells.

2 What are the similarities between bacteria and viruses?

- Some bacteria and viruses can make humans sick.
- People whose immune systems are healthy can successfully fight off many kinds of infections caused by bacteria and viruses.
- There are many kinds of bacteria and viruses that doctors can treat.

3 What is HIV?

4 What kind of cells does HIV mainly infect?

5 What are some of the challenges that scientists face in finding a cure for HIV?

- How do they make a medicine that can tell the difference between infected cells and uninfected cells?

- How do they make a medicine that can kill infected cells without killing uninfected cells?
- How do they find a way to keep HIV from entering white blood cells once HIV is inside the body?

6 How do you feel when you think abut HIV?

Frightened, angry, upset, confident, OK, etc.

7 Is HIV scary?

HIV is scary. It can do very bad things to a person's immune system. However, scientists are trying to find a cure. Also, there are many treatments that help people with HIV live longer and healthier lives. Fortunately, HIV is preventable.

8 Why is HIV prevention important?

At this time, the only way not to have HIV infection is not to get the virus in the first place.

9 How can we prevent HIV?

HIV only harms the human body once the virus has entered the body. Prevention means keeping the virus out of the body.

Part 4: Lesson Extension & Assessment

1 Working individually, students answer the following questions:

- What is a cell? A bacteria? A virus?
- What can bacteria do when they enter the body?
- What does HIV do inside the body?
- Are there medicines that can cure many types of bacterial infections? What are these medicines called? How do they work?
- Is there a cure for HIV? Why or why not?
- How can people prevent HIV and bacterial infections?
- Why is HIV prevention so important?
- How do you feel about HIV?
- Can you prevent HIV?
- What advice would you give your friends about preventing HIV?

2 In small groups, students create posters, models or other types of artistic projects to communicate the information covered in this activity. Students can "block out" their movements at each step of the activity. Accompanying narrative can explain the visual representations. Alternatively, students choreograph a dance piece based on the activity.

3 Students keep a journal of important vocabulary covered in HIV/STD education lessons. Students demonstrate mastery of vocabulary terms through creative writing projects or informative essays.

Guiding Questions

What are some positive health benefits of eliminating the risk of HIV/STD infection?

What are some positive health benefits of reducing the risk of HIV/STD infection?

What public health information is presented on condom boxes and lubricants?

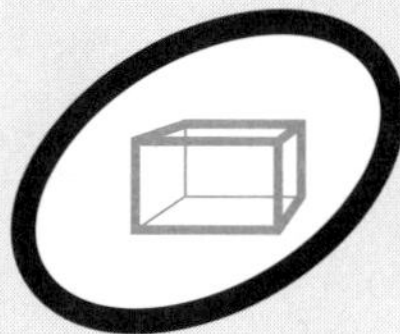

What is the public health role of correct and consistent use of latex condoms for individuals who have chosen/will choose to be sexually active?

Content: Attitudes, Knowledge, Skills

Recommended Grade Level: 8-9

Correlation to Standards: Health Education: 1, 2, 3, 4, 5, 6, 7; Science Education: A, E, F, G

Estimated Time: 25 minutes excluding Lesson Extension & Assessment

Materials: An assortment of condom boxes for lambskin, lubricated latex, spermicidally lubricated latex, non-lubricated latex, polyurethane, female condoms, and novelty condoms. A few boxes of lubricants including water-based spermicidal, water-based non-spermicidal and non-water-based (i.e. petroleum jelly).

Part 1: Learning From the Boxes

1. Distribute the assorted condom boxes and lubricant boxes to the class. Each student may take one to look at during the activity. Students who do not want to hold the boxes can pass.
2. Ask the students to read the information on the condom boxes. Can they find the expiration date or the date of manufacture? Can they locate the disclaimer that explains what the condoms can and cannot do?
3. Ask the students to raise their hands if they have boxes for latex condoms. Have one person read the disclaimer to the class.
4. Ask the students to raise their hands if they have boxes for polyurethane condoms. Have one person read the disclaimer to the class.
5. Ask the students to raise their hands if they have boxes for lambskin condoms. Have one person read the disclaimer to the class.

6 Ask the students to raise their hands if they have boxes for female condoms. Have one person read the disclaimer to the class.

7 Ask the students to raise their hands if they have boxes for novelty condoms. How can you identify novelty condoms? Have one person read the disclaimer to the class.

8 How many students have boxes containing lubricated latex condoms? What does the word "lubricant" tell the consumer about the ingredients used in the product? What is the difference between *specially* lubricated and spermicidally lubricated? What is nonoxynol-9?

9 Ask the students to raise their hands if they have a box containing pure lubricant (not lubricated condoms). Have students read the ingredients and disclaimers for each kind of lubricant.

10 What are condoms designed to do?

> Condoms are designed to prevent one person's sexual fluids from coming into contact with another person's mucous membranes.

11 Do condoms always prevent HIV/STDs and pregnancy?

> No. However, they can prevent HIV, STDs and pregnancy when used correctly and consistently.

12 Discuss the difference between latex or polyurethane condoms and lambskin condoms. Why are latex or polyurethane condoms recommended over lambskin?

> HIV does not pass through intact latex or polyurethane condoms. HIV can pass through the pores in lambskin condoms.

13 Why is the use of a proper lubricant an important step in the correct use of condoms? Why should only water-based lubricants be used with latex condoms? Why is it not a good idea to use oil-based lubricants such as massage oil, moisturizing creams and petroleum jelly? Are all lubricants also spermicides?

> Unlike oil-based lubricants, the water-based lubricants do not damage condoms. Water-based lubricants help prevent the condoms from breaking.

14 Why are disclaimers printed on the condom boxes? What is the purpose of public information?

15 Review the steps involved with correct and consistent use of condoms. See Talking about Condoms with Young Teens.

16 What is the purpose of the female condom?

> It has the same purpose as the male condom.

17 Where can students get condoms?

> Discuss the process of purchasing condoms.

18 Compare and contrast the risk of HIV/STD transmission and pregnancy related to different sexual behaviors using the following questions:

- How much risk is associated with unprotected intercourse?
- How about protected intercourse?
- Is there any risk of HIV infection in a mutually monogamous, trusting relationship, where both partners are HIV negative and have no risk behaviors?
- Why is risk elimination the safest choice?

Lesson Extension & Assessment

1 In small groups, students discuss the importance of communication in risk reduction. Are two partners ready to have sex if they are uncomfortable talking about sex? In contrast, should partners automatically have sex if they can talk openly about protection? Each group creates a skit to express its views. Present skits to the class, and family/community members, if possible.

2 Working in small groups of two or three members, students consider the obstacles and supports related to discussing condom use. Each group creates, practices and demonstrates risk elimination and relevant risk reduction statements.

3 Working in small groups, students research where to buy condoms in their community. Students evaluate different venues for ease of access, selection, and degree of comfort for a young person. Students interview store managers about their experience with selling condoms to young people. Groups present their research in poster or brochure format.

Guiding Questions

How do people make decisions?

Do people make decisions about issues of different importance?

How can people consider the possible outcomes of decisions?

What is the importance of considering options and outcomes with regard to decision making?

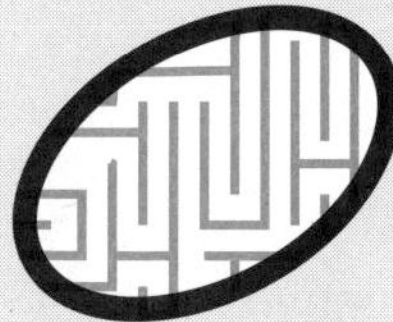

What is the role of sexual decision making in the context of preventing HIV and other STDs?

Content: Attitudes, Skills

Recommended Grade Level: 8-9

Correlation to Standards: Health Education: 1, 3, 4, 5, 6, 7; Science Education: A, F

Estimated Time: 20 minutes excluding Lesson Extension & Assessment

Materials: Writing paper and pen/pencil for each student

Part 1: The Significance of Decisions

1 What is the definition of the word "options?"

Possible choices

2 What is the definition of the word "outcomes?"

What can happen as a result of choosing an option.

3 What was the first decision you made this morning?

Typical responses include the decision to wake up, to take a shower, to eat breakfast, to take the school bus, etc.

4 Did you have any other options?

5 What were the desirable and undesirable outcomes for your decision?

6 What would have happened if you had not made that decision?

7 Did anyone else participate in your decision?

8 How long did it take you to make this decision?

9 How important was this decision in your life?

10 Ask the class if anyone made a really important decision in the past year (such as to change schools, live with a different family member, etc.). Apply the progression outlined above to a few, more important decisions.

11 Ask the class to compare and contrast the decision-making process for choices that are of lesser and greater significance.

Part 2: Sexual Decision Making Discussion

1 Why do people have sex?

2 Why do people not have sex?

3 What is sexual decision making?

The process of choosing what to do with regard to a sexual situation.

4 What is communication?

5 What is the role of communication in sexual decision making?

6 What is the role of personal beliefs in sexual decision making?

7 Why do some people choose to avoid or eliminate all risk of HIV/STD infection?

8 Why do some people choose to reduce the risk of HIV/STD infection?

9 Do students agree or disagree with the following statement? Why or why not?

"If you don't feel comfortable talking about sex with your partner, you're not ready to have sex together. And, if you can talk about sex with your partner, that does not mean you must have sex."

Students often agree with this statement. However, many of these same students will also comment that they think that it is more difficult to have honest communication about sex than to have sex itself. This type of response is an excellent place to begin with a relevant class discussion about the importance of communication in sexual decision making and HIV/STD prevention

10 **Review the following points:**

- People make many decisions every day.
- There are outcomes for all decisions. The impact of different outcomes can range from insignificant to life-changing. The effects of different outcomes can be desirable, neutral or undesirable.
- Outcomes from sexual decision making can have a major effect on a person's health and life experience.
- With regard to sex, the only 100% safe choice is to eliminate the risk of HIV/STD infection.
- However, using condoms can lower the chance of HIV/STD infection if people choose to take the risk of having sex.
- Communication plays an important role in sexual decision making and HIV/STD prevention.

Part 3: Letter to a Friend

1 Students write a letter giving advice to a very close friend (real or imaginary) who is deciding whether or not to have sex.

Lesson Extension & Assessment

1 Review the students' letters from Part 3, Step 1, to assess students' internalization of the activity's main points.

2 In small groups, students brainstorm responses to the following questions:

- What is the meaning of the term *good advice*?
- What is the meaning of the term *bad advice*?
- Do people generally follow the advice they give to other people?
- What makes it easier to take someone else's advice?

Groups use the results from their brainstorming session to make posters entitled "Advice on Advice." Display the posters.

3 Students write a personal essay or journal entry describing their experiences or feelings about giving and receiving advice. Students should explore the following questions:

- Who benefits from good advice — the person to whom the advice is directed, the person giving the advice and/or other people who hear the advice?
- What should a person do if he/she disagrees with someone else's advice?

Guiding Questions

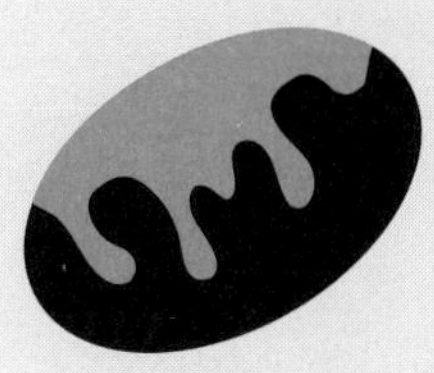

What is the mechanism of HIV infection?

How does the concept of doorways explain the mechanism of HIV infection?

What are developmentally appropriate responses to risky situations?

What are some of the emotional and social factors present in risky situations

Content: Knowledge, Skills

Recommended Grade Level: 5-9

Correlation to Standards: Health Education: 1, 3, 5, 6, 7; Science Education: A, C, E, F, G

Estimated Time: 25 minutes excluding Lesson Extension & Assessment

Part 1: The Concepts of Doorways and Walls

1 What are the body fluids that can transmit HIV and many other STDs?

Blood, sexual fluids (semen and pre-ejaculatory fluid as well as vaginal secretions), and breast milk can transmit HIV and many other STDs.

2 Which body fluids do not transmit HIV or STDs unless mixed with blood, sexual fluids, and/or breast milk?

Saliva, sweat, tears, urine, and mucus from the nose (snot) do not transmit HIV/STDs unless mixed with blood, sexual fluids, and/or breast milk.

3 How does HIV infection happen?

One person's infectious fluids contact another person's blood and/or mucous membranes.

4 How can HIV get into a person's blood?

HIV can get into a person's blood directly through cuts, use of shared needles, or other sharp instruments that have HIV infected blood on them.

5 What is a mucous membrane?

A delicate tissue different from skin which lines some of the openings into the human body.

6 Use your hands to help create a visual image for the following analogy:

> It is dinner time. You're making spaghetti. You have a pot full of hot water and spaghetti. The spaghetti is cooked and will get really mushy unless you get it out of the hot water. What do you do? (Usually, you pour the hot water and the spaghetti through a strainer.) What happens? (Unless you spill everything, the water flows through the strainer while the spaghetti stays inside the strainer.) Why does the water pass through the strainer when the spaghetti does not? (The water is small enough to pass through the holes in the strainer whereas the spaghetti is too big.)

- A mucous membrane is like a strainer.
- HIV is like water.
- Everything else in blood, sexual fluids, and breast milk is like spaghetti.
- When HIV infected blood, sexual fluids, and/or breast milk come into contact with a mucous membrane, the virus can enter white blood cells that are near the surface of the mucous membrane, thereby infecting the body.

7 What are some examples of mucous membranes?

The tissue on the inside of the mouth, eyes, nose, vagina, anus, and opening at the tip of the penis are mucous membranes. The inside of the ear is not a mucous membrane.

8 Everyone should gently pull down their own lower lip and look at each other's lower lip. Ask students to describe what they see. Does this mucous membrane look like skin? Why or why not?

9 What does the term mechanism of transmission mean?

The way transmission occurs.

10 For the purpose of this Activity, imagine that mucous membranes and cuts in the skin are different kinds of doorways into the body. Some mucous membranes are one-way doorways through which HIV can only move in one direction, going into the body;

11 Some mucous membranes are one-way doorways through which HIV can only move in one direction, going into the body. If available, stand by a one-way doorway and demonstrate how the door swings open in one direction only and similarly swings shut in the opposite direction. In the absence of a real example, use your hands to demonstrate this concept.

12 Two-way doorways are places through which HIV can move into and out of the body. If available, stand by a two-way doorway and demonstrate how the door swings open in one direction only and similarly swings shut in the opposite direction. In the absence of a real example, use you hands to demonstrate this concept.

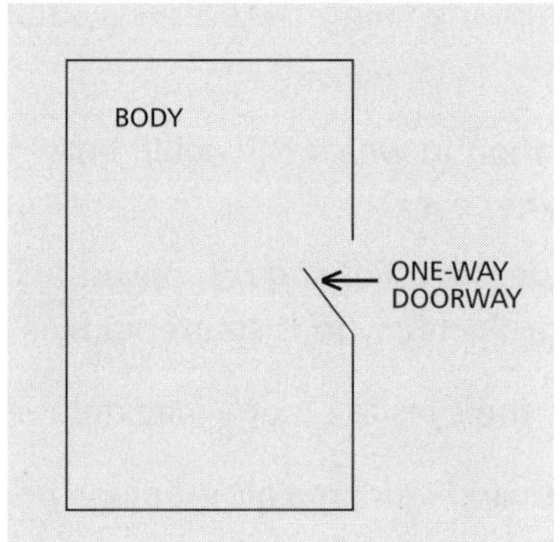

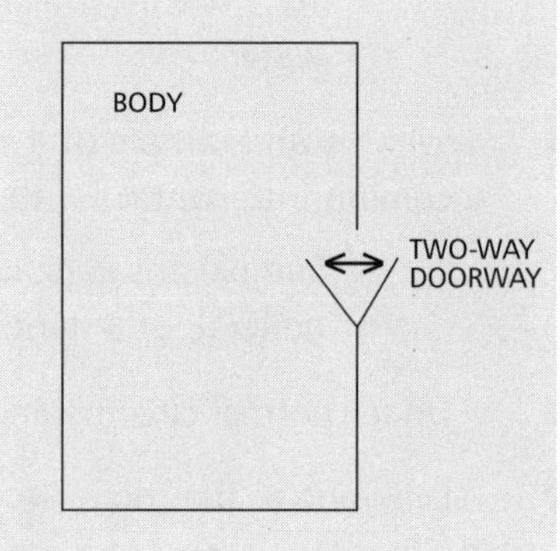

13 Two-way doorways are places through which HIV can move into and out of the body. If available, stand by a two-way doorway and demonstrate how the door swings open and shut in both directions. In the absence of a real example, use your hands to demonstrate this concept. As an example, suggest that students imagine the doorway into a restaurant kitchen.

14 Open cuts are always two-way doorways.

15 The skin is a wall since HIV does not go through intact skin.

16 Point to a wall.

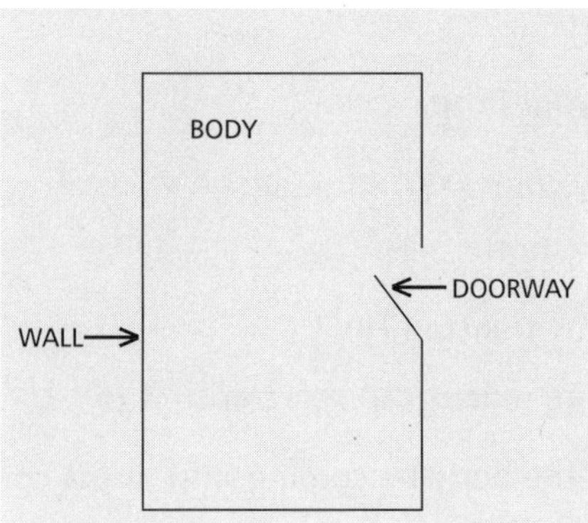

Part 2: One-Way Doorways and Walls

The Eyes

1 Point toward your eyes.

2 What normally comes out of a person's eyes?

Tears.

3 Can pure tears transmit HIV?

No.

4 Can HIV enter the body by coming into direct contact with the mucous membrane lining the eyes? Why?

Yes. The mucous membrane lining the eyes is a strainer and HIV is like water.

5 What is an example of a situation in which HIV could enter a person's body by coming into contact with his/her eyes?

Sample answers include the following responses: first aid situations, in general, or a dentist or doctor who is spattered by a patient's blood.

6 Under normal circumstances, the eyes are a one-way door into the body:

7 Everyone in the room (teacher and students alike) brings both hands up to his/her eyes. (The term "under normal circumstances" means that the eyes are not injured or infected and that there are no other potentially infectious fluids in the eyes.)

8 Everyone waves both hands toward his/her own eyes to indicate how HIV can enter the body in a one-way direction through the eyes.

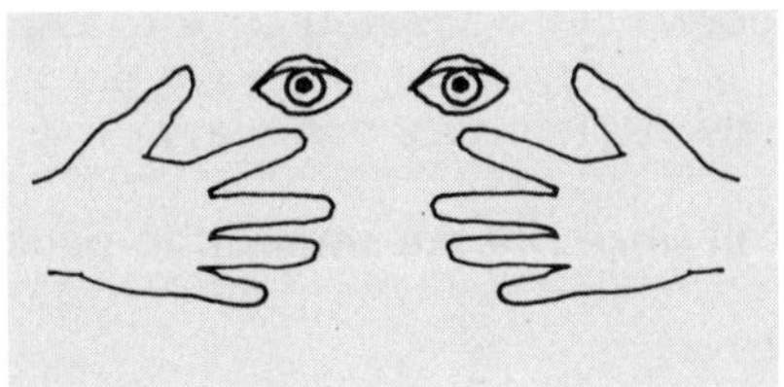

The Nose

1 Point toward your nose.

2 What normally comes out of a person's nose?

Mucus (snot).

3 Can pure mucus transmit HIV?

No. Pure mucus can not transmit HIV.

4 Can HIV enter the body by coming into direct contact with the mucous membrane lining the nose? Why?

Yes. The mucous membrane lining the nose is like a strainer and HIV is like water.

5 What is an example of a situation in which HIV could enter a person's body by coming into contact with his/her nose?

Sample answers include the following responses: first aid situations, in general, or a dentist or doctor who is spattered by a patient's blood or a little kid who gets someone else's blood on his/her finger and then picks his/her nose.

6 Under normal circumstances, the nose is a one-way door into the body.

7 Everyone in the room (teacher and students alike) brings both hands up to his/her nose. (The term "under normal circumstances" means that the nose is not injured or infected and that there are no other potentially infectious fluids in the nose.)

8 Everyone waves both hands toward his/her own nose to indicate how HIV can enter the body in a one-way direction through the nose.

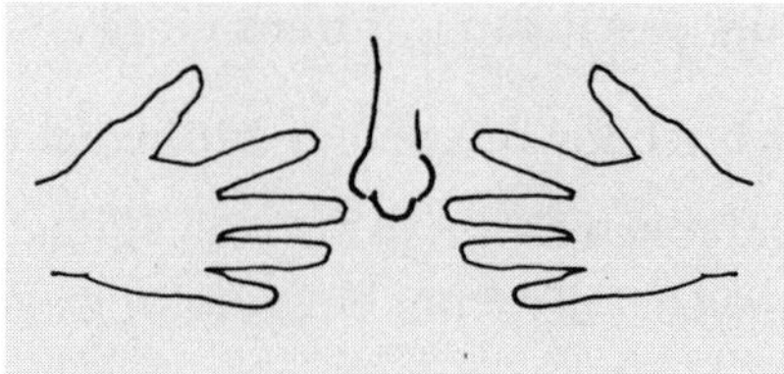

The Mouth

1 Point toward your mouth.

2 What normally comes out of a person's mouth?

Saliva.

3 Can pure saliva transmit HIV?

No. Pure saliva can not transmit HIV.

4 Can HIV enter the body by coming into direct contact with the mucous membrane lining the mouth? Why?

Yes. The mucous membrane lining the mouth is like a strainer and HIV is like water.

5 What is an example of a situation in which HIV could enter a person's body by coming into contact with his/her mouth?

Sample answers include the following responses: a baby drinking HIV infected breast milk, kissing a person who is bleeding, and (if developmentally appropriate) oral sex.

6 Under normal circumstances, the mouth is a one-way door into the body.

7 Everyone in the room (teacher and students alike) brings both hands up to his/her mouth. (The term "under normal circumstances" means that the mouth is not injured or infected and that there are no other potentially infectious fluids in the mouth.)

8 Everyone waves both hands toward his/her own mouth to indicate how HIV can enter the body in a one-way direction through the mouth.

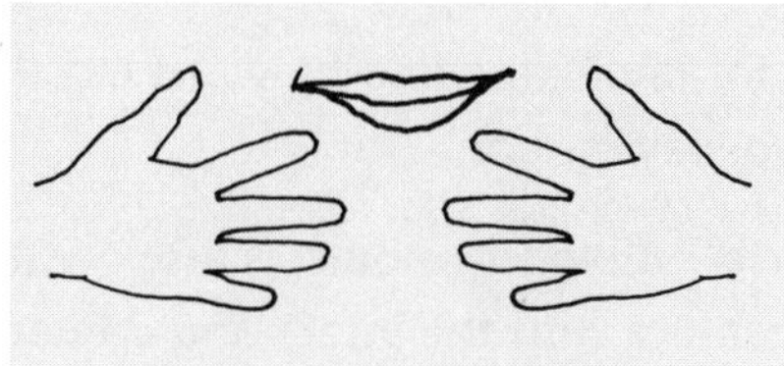

The Skin

1 Point toward your skin

2 What normally comes out of a person's skin?

Sweat.

3 Can pure sweat transmit HIV?

No. Pure sweat can not transmit HIV.

4 Can HIV enter the body by coming into direct contact with the skin? Why not?

No. Unbroken skin is like a wall. Intact skin provides an effective barrier that prevents HIV from entering or exiting a person's body.

5 Under normal circumstances, the skin is a wall.

6 Everyone in the room (teacher and students alike) looks at the intact skin of his/her own hands or arms.

Part 3: Two-Way Doorways — Case Studies

1 Students use their hands to demonstrate the type of doorway (one- way or two-way) presented by the following scenarios:

Bloody nose - A bloody nose is a two-way doorway. HIV can enter the body by coming into contact with the mucous membranes inside the nose and some HIV can exit the body through the blood and bloody mucus leaving the nose during a nose bleed.

Check for understanding by watching the class to see that everyone uses the two-way motion.

Open cut or sore on the skin - An open cut or sore on the skin is a two-way doorway. HIV can enter the body by coming into contact with the open cut or sore on the skin and some HIV can exit the body through the blood coming out of the open cut or sore on the skin.

Check for understanding by watching the class to see that everyone uses the two-way motion.

Injured and bleeding eye - An injured and bleeding eye is a two-way door. HIV can enter the body coming into contact with the intact and damaged mucous membranes of the eye and HIV can exit the body through the blood and bloody tears leaving the injured and bleeding eye.

Check for understanding by watching the class to see that everyone uses the two-way motion.

Bloody mouth - A bloody mouth is a two-way door. HIV can enter the body by coming into contact with the intact and damaged mucous membranes of the mouth and upper throat and HIV can exit the body through the blood and bloody saliva leaving the mouth.

Check for understanding by watching the class to see that everyone uses the two-way motion.

Part 4: Two-Way Doorways — The Penis, Vagina and Anus

NOTE: In the context of HIV transmission, the assumption should be that these body areas act as two-way doorways. The intact mucous membranes of the penis, vagina and anus are all vulnerable to HIV. Urine does not transmit HIV, but the other fluids from these areas (semen, pre-ejaculatory fluid, vaginal secretions and blood) can transmit HIV. (Feces can contain blood and can also transmit other diseases.)

1 Why did we wave our hands to demonstrate types of doorways in this activity?

- To see that everyone understands the concepts.
- To help us remember the concepts by "doing something" as opposed to just "hearing or saying something."
- To help us identify the concepts of doorways and walls with our own bodies. No one can see their own eyes, nose and mouth without the assistance of a mirror, etc.
- So, pointing to these body parts helps make the connection between the idea of a nose and my nose.

2 How can we use the concept of doorways to describe HIV/STD prevention?

- Risk reduction means using barriers designed to close the doorways (For example, BAND-AIDS® make artificial walls, as do latex gloves and condoms.)
- Risk elimination means closing the doorways by avoiding any possibility of contact between the doorways and potentially infectious fluids.

Lesson Extension & Assessment:

1 In small groups, students describe several, hypothetical risky situations. Groups use the idea of doorways to explain how HIV infection can happen and identify useful risk reduction and risk elimination strategies for each situation. Groups select/present one situation to the entire class. The class discusses the importance of knowing how to evaluate the risk of HIV transmission in real-life situations.

As a follow up, students work individually to write a brief, personal response to the following question: "Why do we learn to evaluate the mechanism of HIV transmission in different situations instead of just memorizing a list of "risky behaviors?"

2 In small groups, students develop, practice, and present role plays responding to hypothetical situations that present a risk of HIV transmission. Students should focus on appropriate and culturally relevant situations. Invite family and

community members to attend the final presentations.

3 Students write essays or journal entries addressing the following questions:

- How would you feel about being in a real-life situation where people took measures to prevent HIV transmission?
- How would you feel about being in a real-life situation where people did not respond appropriately to prevent HIV?
- Why would someone not respond appropriately to prevent HIV transmission?
- How would it feel to tell your friend that you need to wear gloves?
- What would you do if you were bleeding and someone else wanted to help you (and touch your open cut) without wearing gloves?
- How is the issue of respect, for self and others, central to HIV prevention?

4 Students design artistic representations of the doorways to show how HIV is and is not transmitted.

Guiding Questions

What is emotional safety? Physical safety?

How do emotional and physical safety relate to HIV/STD prevention?

Why is communication a main component of risk reduction and risk elimination?

What are some developmentally appropriate risk elimination and risk reduction statements?

What are refusal and negotiation skills?

Content: Attitudes, Skills

Recommended Grade Level: 7-9

Correlation to Standards: Health Education: 1, 3, 4, 5, 6; Science Education: A, F, G

Estimated Time: 35 minutes excluding Lesson Extension & Assessment

---

Part 1: Class Discussion

1 What is emotional safety?

Emotional safety means that your feelings are respected, protected, and not in danger.

2 What is physical safety?

Physical safety means that your body is respected, protected, and not in danger.

3 What do the terms emotional and physical safety mean in the context of HIV/STD prevention?

- Emotional and physical safety exist when people are free to decide whether or not to engage in risky behavior; can insist on the use of protection; and respect one another's decisions.

4 Do emotional and physical safety always exist together at the same time? In other words, if you're not safe emotionally, how likely are you to be able to protect yourself physically? If you are safe emotionally, are you automatically safe physically? Could you be safe physically without being safe emotionally?

5 What is the role of communication between sexual partners regarding emotional and physical safety? How does this relate to HIV prevention?

6 How can you know if you're not emotionally or physically safe?

People can have very different responses to danger, but many people know what their own unique cues are. These can include the following: feeling sick to the stomach, feeling choked, getting goosebumps or raised hair on the back of the neck, feeling nervous, trying to justify why the situation isn't unsafe, etc.

7 What can you do if you know that you're not emotionally or physically safe?

Take yourself seriously, figure out what you can do to be safe(r) and do it as soon as possible.

People don't always need to know exactly why they're feeling unsafe. It is more important to make a plan and get to safety as fast as possible; this might mean leaving a specific place, finding other people, or many other strategies.

8 When is it best to address an unsafe situation?

Ideally, it best to **avoid** situations that are emotionally or physically unsafe. But this is not always possible. Many times, situations seem safe, but turn out not to be. Then it is best to respond to feeling unsafe **as soon as you can**. Earlier is almost always better; the longer you wait to "deal" with an unsafe situation, the more unsafe it can get.

9 Can you know if situations are likely to be safe or unsafe?

It is often, but not always, possible to have a good idea about the safety of a situation or activity. There are some helpful things to think about such as:

- Do I know where I'm going and who will be there?
- What do I know about this place and these people?
- What can I do if I want to leave?
- Who knows what I'm doing and where I'll be?
- What do I want to do in this situation?
- What are my feelings about risk and safety? Etc.

10 How do you feel while we're talking about emotional and physical safety?

11 Do you feel as if you can stay safe, emotionally and physically? Would you know what to do if you felt unsafe? What would you do?

12 What does "to refuse" mean? What does "to negotiate," mean? What is a skill?

- To refuse is a verb that means to decline, deny, "say no" or reject something.
- To negotiate is a verb that means to make a deal, create an agreement, or arrange something.
- The word skill is a noun that means the ability to do something well;

usually you have to learn and practice a skill to gain competence or excellence.

13 What are the meanings of the terms refusal and negotiation skills? How could these skills relate to issues of emotional and physical safety?

A person can use refusal skills to "say no" to an unsafe situation. Negotiation skills can help a person make a situation safer. (Teacher models refusal and negotiation skills.)

Part 2: Safety and Sex

1 Ask students to define the terms "emotional safety" and "physical safety."

2 Write, "Why Do People Have Sex?" on the top of the blackboard.

3 Ask students to brainstorm responses to the questions. List students' responses.

4 Discuss which of the reasons on the list are likely to be emotionally safe for both sexual partners. **Circle the students' choices.** Note that some responses may be only partially safe.

5 Discuss which of the reasons are likely to be physically safe for sexual partners. **Underline the students' choices.** Note that some responses may be only partially safe.

6 How many of the circled responses are also underlined? What does this suggest?

7 Which comes first, emotional safety or physical safety? In other words, if you're safe physically are you likely to be able to be safe emotionally and vice-versa? If you're in physical danger how likely are you also to be in emotional danger and vice-versa? Why?

8 Discuss emotionally and physically safe and unsafe reasons why people have sex.

9 Review how people can know if they are in emotional or physical danger.

10 Identify some scenarios in which emotional and physical safety is in question. Discuss the scenarios using the following questions:

- What could students do to negotiate these situations?
- What could they say to ensure their own safety?
- What are the pressures students experience in such situations?
- How can we identify such situations in real life before they happen?
- Do people typically pick up on physical or emotional danger first?
- Discuss the importance of trusting one's instincts that a situation may be dangerous. Also, reinforce the right of each person to be safe(r).

Lesson Extension & Assessment

1. In pairs, students identify realistic scenarios in which they, or their peers, could confront emotionally or physically unsafe situations (including but not limited to situations with the risk of HIV/STD infection). Students work together to create, practice and demonstrate using negotiation and refusal skills that support emotional and physical safety.

2. Students address the issues of emotional and physical safety in other contexts, beyond HIV/STD prevention. For example, in a thematic unit on the law, students research and present findings about the connections between emotional and physical safety and areas covered by the legal system.

Guiding Questions

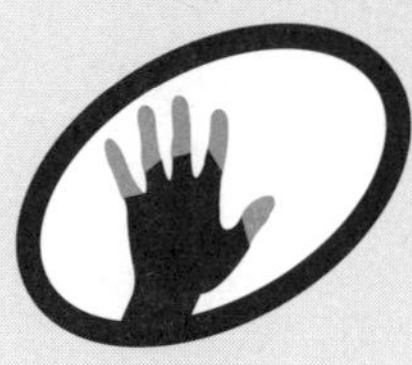

What does the term universal precautions mean?

How do universal precautions apply to HIV/STD prevention?

How are latex gloves used in universal precautions?

What is the right way to use latex gloves?

Content: Attitudes, Skills, Knowledge

Recommended Grade Level: 5-6

Correlation to Standards: Health Education: 1, 3, 4, 5, 6, 7; Science Education: A, C, E, F, G

Estimated Time: 25 minutes excluding Lesson Extension & Assessment

Materials: Three pairs of latex (or vinyl) gloves or one pair of gloves per student*; a variety of colored magic markers; one plastic garbage bag.
(*students with known allergies to latex should not touch latex gloves.)

Part 1: Latex Gloves

1. Distribute pairs of latex gloves to a few students.

2. Students demonstrate the strength and durability of the latex gloves by stretching them. Students put the gloves on their hands.

3. Who in our community wears latex gloves?

   Answers usually include doctors, nurses, firefighters, paramedics and dentists.

4. Why do these people wear latex gloves?

   Doctors, firefighters, paramedics and dentists etc. always wear latex gloves to protect themselves, and the people they are taking care of, from diseases that can be passed through blood. Also, people commonly have germs on their hands that can cause infections in open wounds. Wearing gloves reduces the risk of these infections.

5. What is the definition of the term Universal Precautions?

   Universal precautions is the medical practice of always wearing gloves and/or other protective barriers if there is any chance of contacting some else's body fluids such as blood, sexual fluids, vomit etc.

6. Distribute magic markers of different colors to several of the students who are not

wearing gloves. The magic markers represent blood. Each differently colored magic marker represents a different person's blood. Each person's blood is unique. An uncapped magic marker represents a bloody cut on the hand.

7 Each gloved student approaches a student holding an uncapped magic marker. The gloved student asks permission to provide first aid to the student with the magic marker. With permission, the gloved student puts his/her gloved hands on the magic marker. The student with the marker draws on the first aider's gloves to demonstrate how blood covers the latex glove during first aid.

8 Elect one student with a "bloody glove." This student approaches a "bleeding student" who is holding a different colored marker versus the ink on the first aider's gloves.

9 Can a person who already has "bloody gloves" from one injured person go on to give first aid to another injured student? (In other words, if the gloved student already has orange ink on his/her gloves, is it OK for him/her to give first aid to a student with a blue magic marker?)

No.

- The gloves provide protection both for the first aid provider and the injured person.
- If the first aider provider reuses the gloves to help another injured person, that injured person will be at risk for HIV/STDs (and other blood-borne infections) from contact with the first person's blood. In this case, the first aider is not at risk him/herself.
- The first aider is responsible for his/her own safety and the safety of the injured person.

10 Is it safe for a first aider wearing bloody latex gloves to rub his/her own eyes or an unprotected part of his/her body? Why or why not?

No. By rubbing his/her eyes etc. with bloody gloves, a first aider would have direct contact with someone else's blood.

11 Would an injured person want a first aider to wear gloves? Why or why not?

Yes. Gloves can protect the injured person from the germs/blood that might be present on the first aider's hands.

12 Demonstrate the correct procedure for removing latex gloves by using one gloved hand to grab the other latex glove close to the wrist (without touching the skin), and then pull the glove off, inside-out. Drop the discarded glove into the palm of the gloved hand. Pull the remaining glove inside out over the discarded glove by using the fingers of the bare hand to reach under the wrist opening of the not-yet-discarded latex glove. Then, put the used gloves into the garbage bag.

Ideally, special red biohazard bags would be available for disposal of bloody gloves. However, using garbage bags is more realistic for non-medical settings and provides a better option better than simply throwing used gloves into an open trash container.

13 Students remove their gloves, put the used gloves in the plastic bag, and designate one person to tie the bag shut once all the gloves are inside.

14 Everyone washes his/her hands with soap and warm water after wearing latex gloves. Hand washing is excellent practice for maintaining good hygiene. Hand washing can help reduce the risk of infection if the gloves leaked. Also, many people have skin sensitivities to the powder on the inside of the gloves and to latex itself.

15 Brainstorm with students about where they can get gloves for first aid situations.

Part 2: Class Discussion

1 What does the term personal responsibility mean?

2 Do individuals in a community have the personal responsibility to help an injured person?

3 What are some safe ways to help an injured person who is bleeding?

Responses can include: wearing gloves to apply first aid; calling an ambulance/getting an adult while comforting the injured person; bringing first aid supplies to the injured person; and instructing him/her how to use them.

4 When should you get professional help?

Responses should address the difference between serious injuries and minor injuries. For example, life-threatening situations require more than first aid, so getting an ambulance is more useful than getting gloves.

Lesson Extension & Assessment:

1 In small groups or as an individual assignment, students create posters that communicate the correct procedures for using latex gloves.

2 In small groups or as an individual assignment, students create a skit in which they mime the process of using latex gloves correctly. (Mime = demonstrate without using sounds/words.)

3 In small groups, students brainstorm responses for the following questions:

- Would you wear gloves to help a stranger who was bleeding?
- Would wearing gloves with a stranger be disrespectful?
- Would you wear gloves to help a friend who was bleeding?
- Would wearing gloves with a friend be disrespectful?
- Is there a difference in risk of HIV/STD transmission between these two scenarios?
- Is wearing gloves a sign of respect? Why or why not?
- How could a first aider explain the reasons for practicing universal precautions in a comfortable and appropriate way regardless of

whether the injured person is a friend or a stranger?

4 Students write an essay or a journal entry addressing the following situation:

Imagine that you are bleeding. How would you feel if someone tried to help you without wearing gloves? Do you have the right to tell the person to go get gloves, call for help, etc., and not touch you with his/her bare hands? How would you ask/tell someone to wear gloves in this situation?

If developmentally appropriate, discuss other latex barriers such as condoms and address the following questions:

- Are these barriers designed to function in the same manner as gloves?

  Yes.

- What are condoms designed to do?

  Condoms are designed to function as barriers in the same manner as latex gloves.

- Who are condoms designed to protect?

  Like gloves, condoms are designed to protect both people.

- Who is responsible for using barriers to reduce the risks associated with sexual behaviors?

  Both people involved in sexual behaviors are responsible for using barriers to reduce their risks.

- Are any latex barriers (gloves, condoms etc.) 100% safe?

  Latex barriers are never 100% safe.

- Is there typically a difference in risk level between using a glove during first aid and using condoms during sexual intercourse?

  There is a greater risk associated with using condoms during sexual intercourse than using gloves in a first aid situation. Typically, only the injured person is bleeding in a first aid situation and the skin on the first aider's hand provides protection against HIV/STDs in the event of a broken glove. In contrast, during sexual intercourse, both people can be exposed to each other's sexual fluids in parts of both of their bodies that are vulnerable to HIV/STDs. So, if the condom breaks there is a high-risk for both partners.

- What does this mean in terms of decision making about first aid and also, about sex?

  With regard to first aid situations, we have the responsibility to seek appropriate help for an injured person — whether we wear gloves to provide the care directly or call for medical assistance. With regard to sexual behaviors, the safest choice is to wait to have sex until we are in a safe relationship where both people are free of HIV/STDs (based on test results), have no other risk factors for HIV/STDs, and share trust, communication, respect and commitment.

Guiding Questions

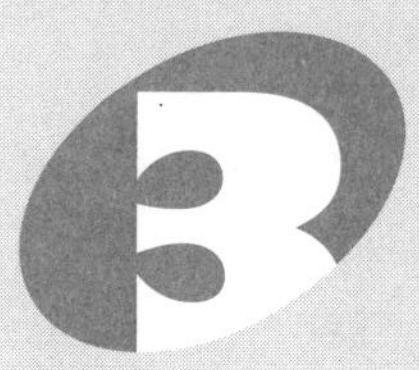

What is the HIV antibody test and how does it work?

What is the importance of the three month window period in HIV testing?

What are different people's attitudes regarding use of the HIV antibody test?

Content: Knowledge, Attitudes

Recommended Grade Level: 7-8

Correlation to Standards: Health Education: 1, 3, 4, 5, 6, 7; Science Education: A, C, E, F, G

Estimated Time: 25 minutes excluding Lesson Extension & Assessment

Set Up: Sufficient open space for seven to twelve students to stand in a line, shoulder to shoulder, facing the class.

Part 1: Activity

1 What does the HIV antibody test actually show?

The HIV antibody test is a blood test that identifies the antibodies to HIV, which will, almost always, be detectable in a person's blood three months after HIV infection.

NOTE: There are now oral and urine tests for HIV. However, these tests are less widely used and are typically more expensive. Therefore, this activity will focus on the HIV antibody blood test. This activity uses the term "HIV test" instead of HIV antibody test to be consistent with common usage.

2 Is the HIV test a test for AIDS?

No.

3 Is the HIV test accurate regardless of when it is conducted?

No. Each person's immune system responds to HIV infection by making antibodies sometime within the three month period after infection. This three month period is commonly called a "window period."

A **negative test** result means that no HIV antibodies were detected. A negative result can be trusted three months after a possible exposure to HIV. At that point, a negative test means that the person does not have HIV (unless infected during the prior three months).

A **positive test** result means that HIV antibodies were detected and (in most cases) the person has HIV infection. Exceptions can include people who received "false-pos" results and babies born to HIV infected moms.

4 How long can it take for the HIV antibodies to become detectable after HIV infection?

It can take up to three months, although it is very common for HIV antibodies to be detectable much sooner after HIV infection.

5 Recruit seven to ten student volunteers. These students line up, standing shoulder to shoulder, facing the class.

6 Working from left to right, assign each student a month (January, February, etc.) so that the line represents consecutive months.

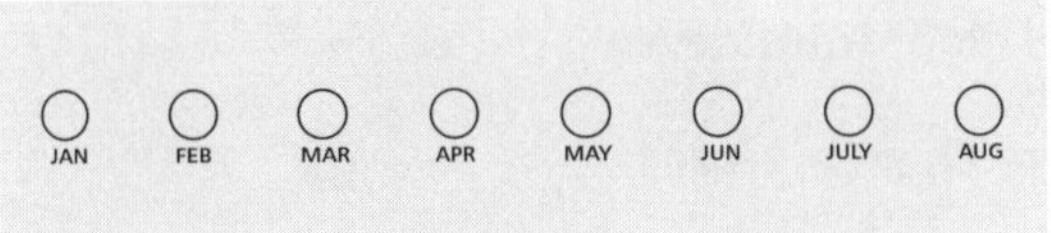

7 Recruit another student to represent the HIV antibodies.

8 The class identifies a hypothetical scenario in which someone engages in a high-risk behavior during January.

9 Build on the hypothetical scenario by informing the class that the person in the scenario decides to get an HIV test because he/she is worried about what happened in January. Before January, this person had no risk of HIV infection.

10 In the scenario, the worried person takes an HIV test in January.

11 Explain that the class can conduct the HIV test for this hypothetical person. The test is a visual test, and the class looks at the line of students representing the months to see when the HIV antibodies are detectable.

12 The student representing HIV antibodies (hereafter the "HIV Antibody") hides (as much as possible) behind the student representing the month of January. Can the class see the HIV Antibody in January? Why not?

No. It is highly unlikely that HIV antibodies would be detectable in the person's blood only weeks after possible infection. If the person is not HIV infected, there will be no antibodies anyway.

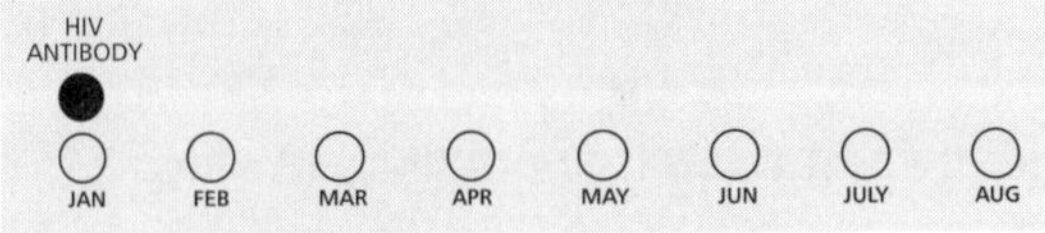

13 The HIV Antibody moves down the line, and hides behind February and then March. Can the class see the HIV Antibody yet? Why not?

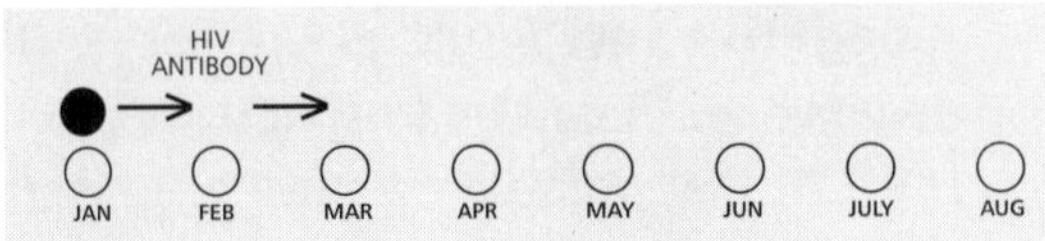

No, even if the person is HIV infected, the HIV antibodies may not yet be detectable by the test. If the person is not HIV infected, there will be no antibodies anyway.

14 The HIV Antibody stands up tall behind (or beside) April so that the class can see the HIV antibody. Can the class see the HIV Antibody now? What does it mean that the class **can** see the HIV Antibody?

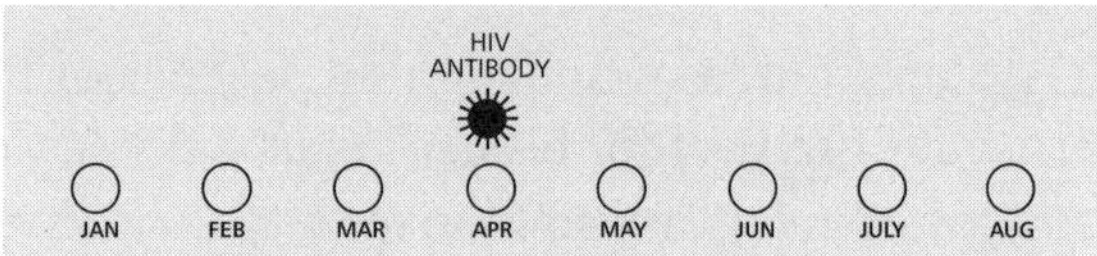

If the class can see the HIV Antibody it means that the person in the hypothetical scenario is HIV positive and has the virus.

15 What would it mean if the class still couldn't see the HIV Antibody in April?

If the class cannot see the HIV Antibody three months after the possible exposure, it means that the person in the hypothetical scenario is HIV negative and does not have the virus unless he or she engaged in another risky behavior since January.

16 Refer to the student representing March. Imagine that the person had engaged in risky behaviors again in March.

17 Would the HIV antibody test done in April be accurate for the hypothetical person if he/she had another potential exposure to HIV in March?

No, it is too soon. The person would need to wait until three months later until June.

The HIV Antibody demonstrates the correct response by moving down the line and stands visibly behind or beside the person representing June.

Part 3: Class Discussion

1 What do you need to know in order to evaluate another person's statement that he/she just had an HIV test and tested negative?

- When did the person have the test?
- Did the person have any possible risks for HIV transmission within a three month period before taking the test?
- Has the person had any possible risks since taking the test?
- How do you know you can trust the person?

2 What are some of the emotional and physical implications of **not knowing** if you have HIV?

3 What are some of the emotional and physical implications of **knowing** that you do have HIV?

4 What are some of the emotional and physical implications of **not knowing** if someone else has/does not have HIV?

5 What are some of the emotional and physical implications of **knowing** that someone else has/does not have HIV?

6 Why/when would someone need/want to take an HIV test?

7 Does a person need to get a test if he/she has never had any risk of HIV transmission?

Sometimes a person with no past risk of HIV infection chooses to get a test out of respect for his/her sexual partner. In such a case, the decision to get tested is less a medical necessity than an emotional issue.

8 Should two virgins get HIV tests before having sex or getting married?

Yes, the only way to be sure that both people are healthy is to take the HIV test. People who are virgins have not had sexual intercourse and could not have become infected with HIV in that way. However, there are many other ways to get infected with this virus. Taking the test together can be a gesture of respect and commitment.

9 Why is it important to determine a person's HIV infection **earlier** as opposed to later?

A person who is HIV positive can begin treatment as soon as possible. HIV prevention remains a major priority — both to prevent transmission to other people and to prevent re-infection from another HIV positive person.

10 Does a person have the right to ask a potential sexual partner to take an HIV test?

Yes, each person has that right. But the law is not the issue here; rather, sexual partners need to communicate their needs to each other and be respectful.

11 Discuss the roles of trust and communication in disease prevention.

12 Discuss appropriate and inappropriate uses of the HIV test. Is it more important for a person to get tested frequently or to change behaviors that put him/her at risk? Why?

13 What might be some of the implications of a negative HIV test result on a person's behavior? What about a positive test?

14 Discuss the implications of HIV testing regarding pregnancy. Is it a good idea for a pregnant woman to take an HIV test? What happens if a pregnant woman tests positive for HIV? Is it a good idea to take the test before the pregnancy? What about the father-to-be? Why?

15 Is it important to have support during the HIV testing process? Would it be a good idea for people to speak with their families and friends about the choice to have a test?

16 What are the pros and cons of mandatory testing? Who currently does mandatory testing? (Sample responses can include the following: the U.S. Military, Job Corps, and Peace Corps.) Could mandatory testing provide a false sense of security? What are the financial, logistical, and civil rights implications of mandatory testing? What about mandatory HIV testing before marriage?

17 What is the role of HIV testing in HIV prevention?

Lesson Extension & Assessment

1 In small groups, students work in the local community to research (some or all of) the questions listed below. Groups develop oral presentations as well as written/artistic supplements to present/display their research findings. Groups present their research findings to the entire class and parents, whenever possible.

- Where can a person go to get an HIV test in the local area?
- What is the testing procedure at the local HIV test site?
- How much does the test cost?
- Who can go in and take a test?
- How long does it take to get the results back?
- Does the local HIV test site offer services specifically designed for adolescents? What are these services?
- Does the local HIV test site offer confidential and/or anonymous HIV testing?
- Compare and contrast confidential and anonymous HIV testing.
- Does the local HIV test site offer pre- and post-test counseling?
- What is the purpose of pre- and post-test counseling?

2 Individually or in small groups, students design their version of adolescent-specific pre- and post-test counseling. Students design role plays to showcase their counseling strategies using hypothetical scenarios.

3 Invite an HIV test counselor to class. Students develop characters who decide to take an HIV test. Students role play with the counselor using their characters' personal stories, attitudes, etc. The role plays demonstrate the non-judgmental, health focus of pre- and post-test counseling.

4 Individually or in small groups, students research the topic of antibodies and immunity. For example, are there different kinds of vaccines that have different effects on antibody production? Students present their work in written, oral, artistic, dramatic, or other creative formats.

5 In small groups, students create action plans for a person who wants to know if he/she has HIV (or similar HIV/STD related question/concern). An action plan answers the questions "who, what, where, when, why, how and what's next" for a specific situation.

(see next page for Action Plan Model)

Action Plan Model:

Sample Action Plan:

- **Who** has the question/concern?

  I do.

- **What** is the question/concern?

  I want to know if I have HIV.

- **Why?**

  I learned about HIV transmission and I have done some risky things. It would be good to know what to do if I have HIV or how to make sure I stay healthy if I don't have HIV.

- **How** can I find out if I have HIV?

  I can go get tested.

- **Where?** And **When?**

  I can use the "Yellow Pages," other public information and/or personal interviews to access information about testing centers. I can call the test center and find out when I can go in for an HIV test.

- **What's next?**

  I can make another action plan to help me get to the clinic, etc.

Guiding Questions

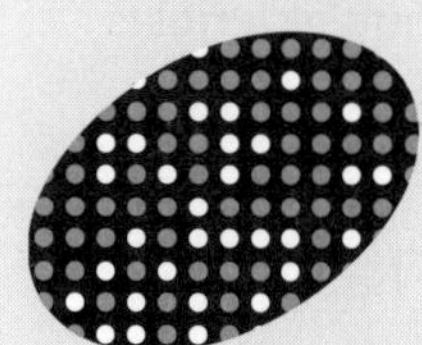

How does HIV mutate during replication?

Is there a connection between HIV mutation and challenges to finding a cure for HIV?

What is the relationship between HIV mutation and HIV prevention?

Why is HIV prevention important?

Content: Knowledge, Attitudes

Recommended Grade Level: 6-7

Correlation to Standards: Health Education: 1, 4; Science Education: A, C, E, F, G

Estimated Time: 35 minutes excluding Lesson Extension & Assessment

Set Up: Create an open space in the classroom.

Part 1: HIV Mutation

1. What does the word **mutation** mean?

   Mutation is a noun that means a change from the parent type so that the next generation has a different (genetic) design.

2. Does HIV mutate? How?

   Yes, HIV often mutates when it replicates. The activity demonstrates this phenomenon.

3. Students stand shoulder-to-shoulder in two equal parallel lines, facing each other. If there are more than twenty students, either use volunteers to demonstrate the activity or break into two sub-groups to complete the activity.

4. One line represents HIV. The other line represents a cure for HIV.

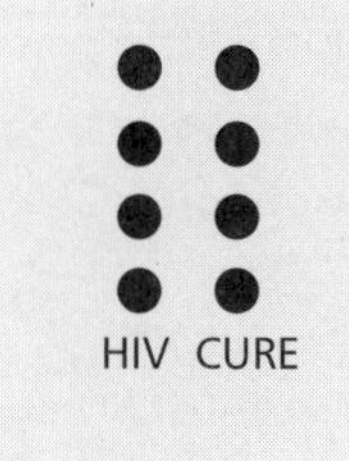

5 Begin with the person at one end of the HIV line. This person holds out one hand and makes a shape with it. This shape can be as complicated or as simple as the person chooses. The shape represents the genetic material of one HIV virus.

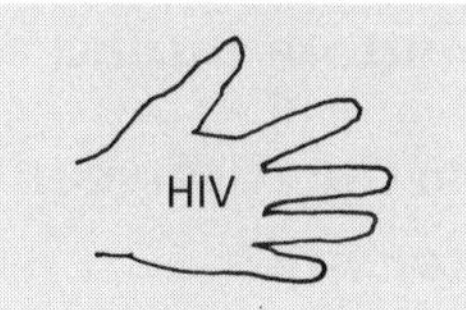

6 Explain that to develop a cure for HIV, or slow down the rate of infection, scientists need to find a substance that can recognize HIV precisely, attach to the virus, and neutralize or destroy it.

7 The person in the cure line opposite the first HIV creates a shape with his/her own hand to match the "HIV virus."

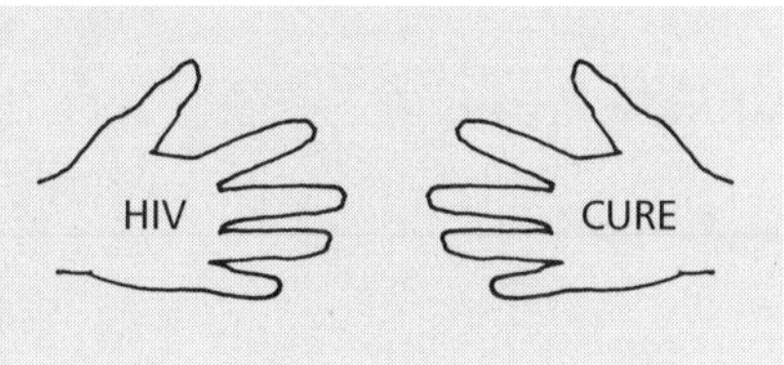

8 The cure matches the HIV.

9 The first HIV shows the next person in the HIV line how to make the original hand shape representing the virus.

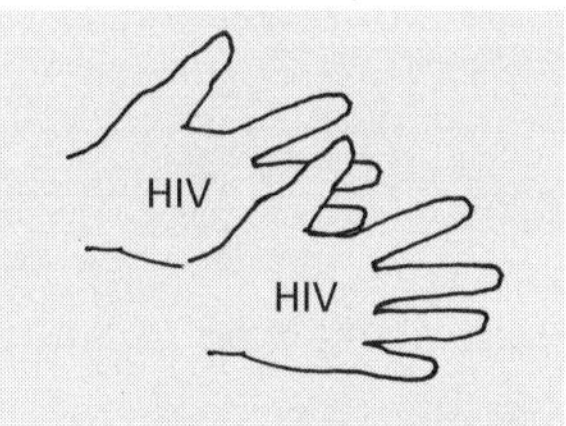

10 The first cure shows the next person in the cure line how to make the original hand shape representing the cure.

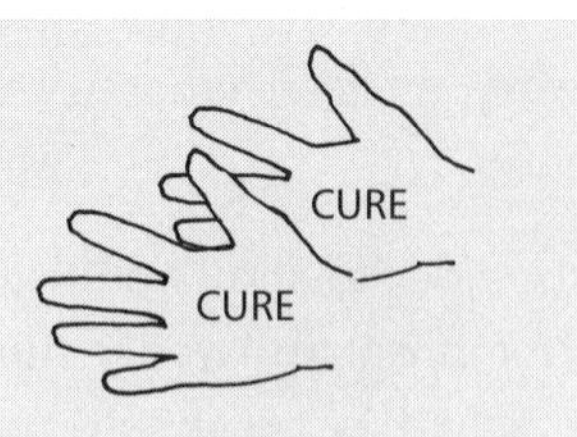

11 The second person in the HIV line makes the original shape and then changes his/her hand shape to represent how HIV mutates when it replicates. This person's hand still represents HIV; however, the second-generation virus should be slightly different from the first generation.

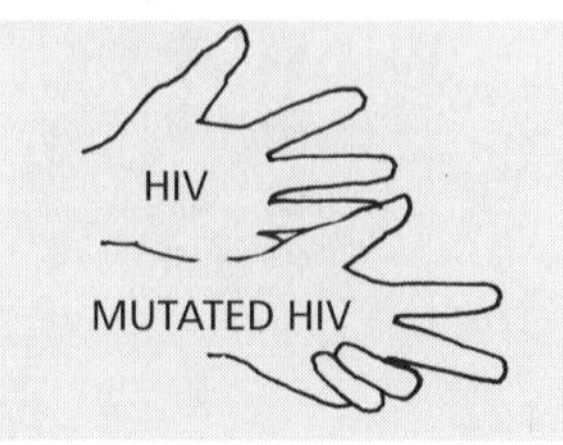

12 The second person in the cure line tries match the first cure to the mutated, second-generation virus. Is it a perfect match? If so, move on to step 13. If not, instruct the second person in the cure line to make a new hand shape to match the mutated virus.

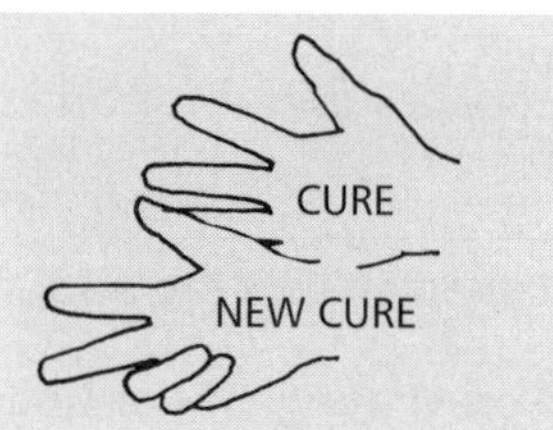

13 Repeat steps 9 - 12 until all of the students in the lines have participated.

14 What happened to the HIVs?

Each version of HIV mutated.

15 Can HIV mutate within one person over time?

Yes.

16 If two people have HIV, and they exchange blood or other infectious fluids can they give each other different versions of HIV?

Yes, and this could harm their health.

17 What happened in the cure line?

The cures had to make adjustments to match the HIV mutations.

18 How well did the cures match the viruses?

Pretty well.

19 Was it easier and faster to make a mutated virus or develop a cure?

It is easier and faster for HIV to mutate than to keep developing new cures.

20 Did the cure line need to keep upgrading the cures to match new viral mutations?

Yes.

21 Would any of the cures work against all of the viruses?

Probably not.

22 What kinds of challenges related to mutation do scientists face in trying to develop a cure or preventative vaccine for HIV?

It is complicated to make a cure that can recognize all of the HIV's mutations but does not harm anything other than HIV. Also, sometimes the mutations are resistant to the medicines used to treat HIV. This means that those medicines stop working well, and a person needs new medicines. In addition, mutations happen very, very quickly whereas it can take years to develop new, safe, and effective medications.

23 Many people working on the development of a cure think that HIV mutation is very interesting. Do the students think doing research on HIV might be interesting and frustrating? Why? Is the process of finding a cure for HIV relatively simple or complicated?

24 What are the kinds of personal qualities that a successful scientist needs in order to do research on a cure for HIV?

Patience, curiosity, tenacity (not giving up), creativity, diligence (sticking to it), knowledge (education) etc.

25 Are these characteristics useful for other people too? How about for students? Why?

26 Which of these characteristics are also important for HIV prevention?

27 Which is simpler: preventing HIV or finding a cure for the virus?

Lesson Extension & Assessment

1 Students make posters that explain how HIV mutates and illustrate the kind of variation possible during mutation.

2 What are other examples of genetic mutation in science? What are some examples of mutations that are beneficial? How about mutations that are harmful?

Guiding Questions

How does HIV replicate?

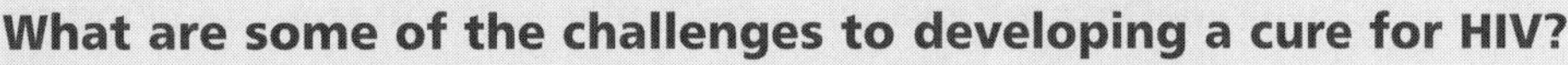

How does HIV effect the human immune system?

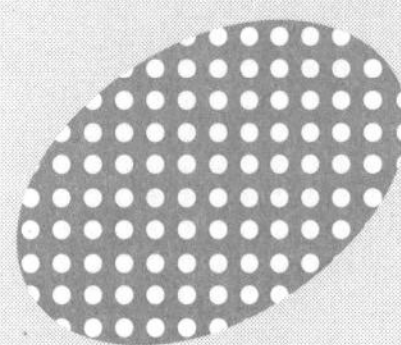

What are some of the challenges to developing a cure for HIV?

Why is HIV prevention important?

Content: Knowledge, Attitudes

Recommended Grade Level: 6-7

Correlation to Standards: Health Education: 1, 4; Science Education: A, C, E, F, G

Estimated Time: 35 minutes excluding Lesson Extension & Assessment

Set Up: An open space sufficient for students to form a large circle by standing together shoulder to shoulder. One freestanding chair per peron.

Part 1: The Shape of HIV

1 Ask the students to form a circle by standing shoulder to shoulder facing inward toward the center of the circle.

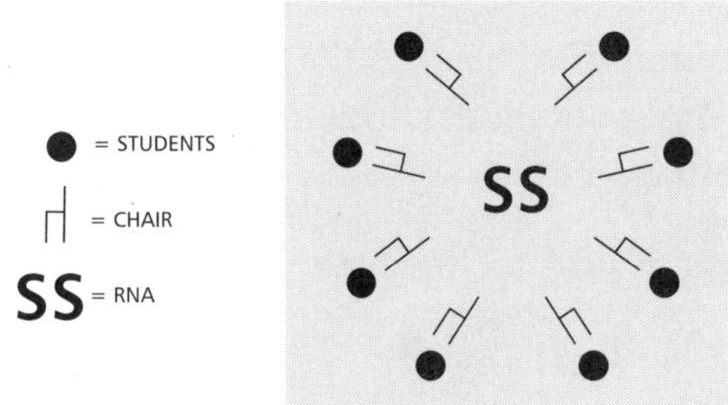

2 Direct the students to arrange the chairs along the circumference of the circle they just created:

The chairs should be positioned so that the back of the chair is lying on the floor with the seat pointing vertically upward and the legs pointing outward from the circle. Students stand outside the circle of chairs.

3 Explain that HIV is a sphere. Imagine that the class has sliced a tiny, pure HIV virus in half and the chairs represent the flat section cut through the virus.

Ask for two volunteers to go to the center of the circle and lie down on their sides, with their knees bent forward so that each person's position is an S-shape. These students represent the two strands of RNA that contain HIV's genetic coding.

Part 2: HIV Encounters a White Blood Cell

1 Focus the class' attention on the chair legs pointing out of the circle. Explain that these legs represent the proteins on the outside of HIV. They are like keys that reach out to join in a lock that is also formed by proteins, called CD-4 receptors, on the outside surface of white blood cells (WBC). WBCs have these locks to enable the cells to fuse with organisms that invade the body. Once attached the WBCs usually destroy the invader or capture it for another white blood cell to kill.

2 Using your arms, demonstrate how the CD-4 receptors (lock) try to grab onto the HIV (keys) by attempting to grab hold of the legs on a few chairs. Finally, grip one set of chair legs tightly to show how the WBC attaches to HIV.

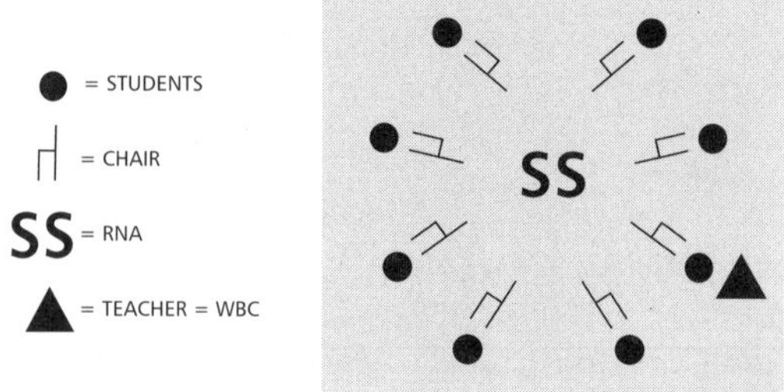

3 Explain that the WBC attaches to HIV as part of the cell's normal immune functioning. In effect, the cell expects to capture and/or destroy the virus. However, HIV has the ability to sabotage the normal process. Once HIV joins with the WBC the virus moves into the cell both to hide from the body's immune system and also to begin to replicate or reproduce itself. Viruses need to inhabit host cells in order to produce more viruses.

Part 3: An HIV Infected White Blood Cell

1 Ask students to reposition the chairs so that the legs are on the ground in the conventional style. The seats should now face into the circle. This new position symbolizes the HIV infected WBC.

2 Direct the two strands of RNA to stand up.

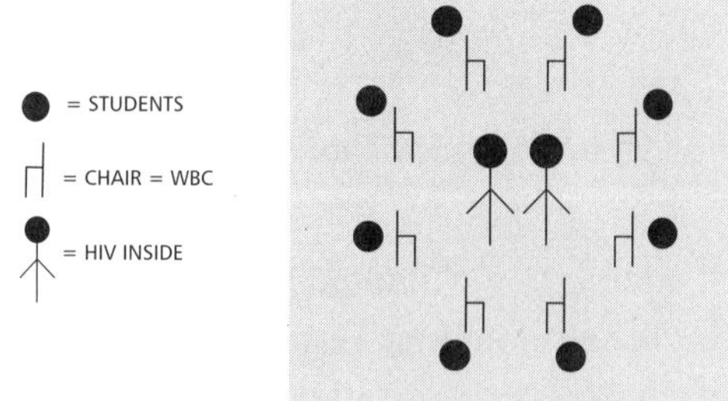

3 Explain that RNA from the HIV is able to integrate into the genetic material of the infected cell. So when the infected cell divides, the virus uses the cell's replication mechanism to produce more viruses.

4 Move all of the students into the center of the circle. The students now represent newly formed HIV particles that have been manufactured by the infected WBC.

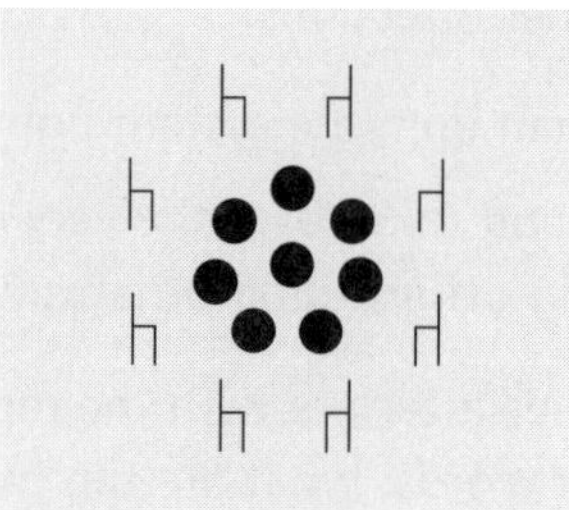

5 Could the entire class fit inside the circle?

6 Would another hundred or thousand new viral particles (students) also fit?

No.

7 What would happen if there were another thousand particles (students) within the circle?

The circle (WBC) would explode, which is exactly what ultimately happens to the infected WBC.

8 What happens to the circle (WBC) when it explodes?

The WBC dies.

However, before exploding, small amounts of HIV start to escape from the cell in a process called budding. Demonstrate this process by asking few students in the circle (cell) to move outside of the circle (cell).

9 All of the students (viral particles) within the cell explode out of the circle.

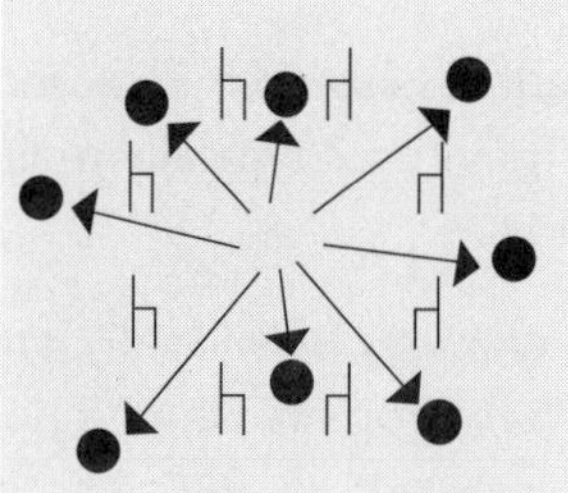

10 Explain that each of the escaped viral particles is capable of starting the entire process all over again in another WBC. In this way HIV manages to undermine the immune system by invading and controlling the very cells whose primary function is to fight off foreign agents in the body. Not only does HIV take over the WBCs, but the virus uses cells to manufacture more viruses, ultimately destroying more and more WBCs in the process.

Part 4: Class Discussion

1 Review the steps necessary for HIV replication: HIV must attach to the cell, penetrate the cell membrane, integrate viral genetic material into the WBC's DNA and ultimately direct the WBC to produce more HIV.

2 How does HIV weaken the human immune system?

> HIV weakens the immune system by killing WBCs so that the body cannot fight off other infections.

3 Why can't the human immune system fight off HIV?

> HIV infects and takes over the very cells that would otherwise be charged with fighting off invading organisms.

4 How could medicines interfere with the replication process to slow down HIV infection? In other words, what are the points in the replication process where the chain of events could be stopped?

> Possible vulnerable points include where HIV attaches to the WBC and when HIV starts to make more of itself inside the WBC.

5 Is the HIV replication process frightening? What can we do about our fears of HIV infection?

> It is natural to be frightened by HIV. One frightening aspect of HIV infection is that the virus seems to be in control once it is inside a person's body. Healthy fear can motivate us to prevent HIV. If we don't let HIV into the body, the virus cannot be in control.

6 Discuss the importance of HIV prevention.

Lesson Extension & Assessment

1 In small groups, or working individually, students research the replication process of other microorganisms. Compare and contrast these other processes with HIV.

2 In small groups, students research RNA and DNA. What kinds of organisms have RNA? DNA? How do viruses typically replicate? Students build models and present their findings.

3 In small groups, or working individually, students research population growth and limiting factors. What happens when a population runs out of food? What happens when HIV runs out of WBCs in a person's body? What kinds of diseases are the most likely to cause long term damage to humans: those that kill their hosts quickly like Ebola or those that kill slowly like HIV? Why? Students present their findings.

4 Students design artistic representations to document HIV replication.

5 Students choreograph a dance documenting HIV replication.

Guiding Questions

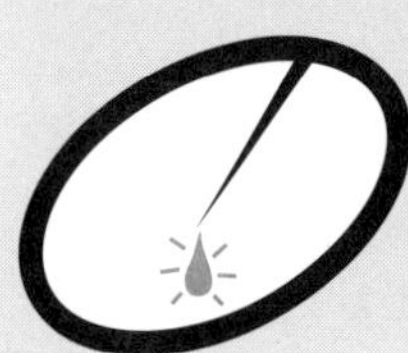

What are the characteristics and effects of common illegal drugs and alcohol?

How can use of illegal substances be directly and indirectly related to the risk of HIV/STD transmission?

Why is avoidance of illegal substances a healthy decision?

Content: Attitudes, Knowledge

Recommended Grade Level: 8-9

Correlation to Standards: Health Education: 1, 2, 5, 7; Science Education: A, C, E, F, G

Estimated Time: 35 minutes excluding Lesson Extension & Assessment

Materials: Research Questions Handout; poster paper and markers.

Part 1: Research

NOTE: Before beginning this activity reinforce the message that the use of alcohol is illegal for people under the age of 21 and legal for adults over the age of 21. All the other drugs discussed here are illegal for everyone. Using these drugs can have serious legal as well as health consequences.

1 Ask participants to list the types of commonly used legal and illegal drugs, highlighting those that are more likely to be used in the local community. Drugs that should be mentioned include the following: alcohol, hallucinogens, cocaine/crack, amphetamines, ecstasy, PCP, and steroids. See Information on Alcohol and Other Drugs.

2 Discuss each of these substances briefly including the type of drug, its effects, whether it is legal or illegal, and the potential long-term effects — such as addiction, withdrawal and health concerns associated with continued use.

3 Students divide into small groups.

4 Assign each group the topic of one of the illegal substances listed above. Be sure to cover: alcohol, marijuana/hashish, ecstasy, cocaine and crack, steroids, and heroin.

5 Each group researches and analyzes its assigned substance according to the criteria on the Research Questions Handout.

(see next page for Research Questions Handout)

Research Questions Handout

- Why do people use this drug?
- What kinds of pressure are there on people to use this drug? Where does this pressure come from? How is the pressure communicated?
- When, where and how is the drug typically used?
- What are some stereotypes about people who use this drug?
- How can people behave when they are using this drug?
- What can people think they gain from using the drug?
- What can people jeopardize or lose by using this drug? What are the potential legal consequences of using this drug?
- How could use of this drug contribute to behaviors that put a person at risk for HIV/STD transmission?

6 Small groups present their research findings and analysis to the class.

Part 2: Class Discussion

1 Are there common themes among the groups' research findings and analysis? What are the similarities? Are there differences among the findings?

Focus on issues of judgment, motivation and priorities, from social acceptance to the symptoms of addiction — e.g. getting the drug now may be more important than being healthy ten years from now.

2 Are there connections between drugs and risk of HIV/STD transmission? See chapter on Information on Alcohol and Other Drugs.

3 What are the direct and indirect routes of HIV transmission associated with injection drug use? See Information on Alcohol and Other Drugs.

4 Discuss students' responses to the following statements:

"Sex feels better when I'm drunk or high."

Alcohol is a depressant, so why do people say that sex feels better when they're drunk?

"I feel more confident when I'm drunk."

Does a person really want to have sex if he/she needs to be high or drunk to do it?

5 Discuss inhibitions and avoidance of conscience. Are people able to make their best decisions while they are drunk?

"It is harder to say 'no' to sex when I'm drunk or high."

Being drunk or high is sometimes used as a justification for having sex irresponsibly. People may say that "it just happened." That way, they avoid having to be responsible for their actions. However, aren't they still responsible for their actions? And aren't they still going to have to deal with the consequences? If it is harder to say 'no,' won't it also be harder to insist on using protection? And won't it be harder to be sure of your physical safety?

"I'm not going to be alive in ten years so why should I worry about HIV now?"

This is a difficult issue to discuss since it is important to address underlying issues of hopelessness and helplessness. However, people often have at least one person in their life whom they want to shield from pain. This might be a grandparent, or a child, or a best friend. Wouldn't dying from AIDS hurt this person? Is it worth it to stay healthy for him/her?

6 Which are more scary, the direct or the indirect connections between substance use and risk of HIV/STD transmission? Why?

7 Can a person eliminate the risk of HIV/STD infection by choosing not to use alcohol and drugs?

> If a person does not use alcohol or other drugs, he/she won't get HIV/STD while using them. And, being sober can definitely help a person avoid risky situations. However, people can be at risk for HIV/STDs from other behaviors that do not involve illegal substances.

8 Why is it a healthy choice to avoid illegal substances?

Lesson Extension & Assessment

1 In small groups, students develop the progression for a short story that examines the direct and indirect connections between substance use and HIV/STD infection. Groups divide the story line into equal length segments and assign a segment to each student. Each student individually writes his/her segment. Groups present their stories by reading the segments aloud to the entire class. Discuss theme development, consistency and inconsistency among segments. Compare and contrast the stories to real life.

2 In small groups or working individually, students design HIV-related public service announcements (PSAs) and advertisements discouraging drug and alcohol use. Present or display students' work. Network with local health clinics and doctors' offices to find display space for students' work for community viewing.

3 In small groups, students design an alcohol and drug prevention curriculum appropriate for students in a lower grade. Students present the curriculum as part of a cross-age teaching initiative. Students produce written descriptions of their experiences with curriculum development and implementation.

4 Which are more scary, the direct or the indirect connections between substance use and risk of HIV/STD transmission? Why?

Guiding Questions

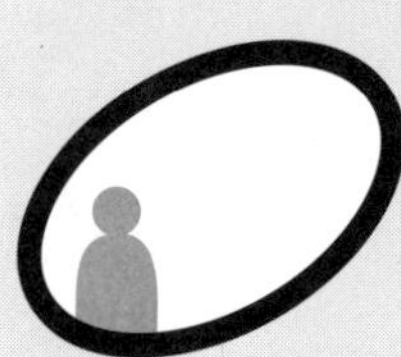

What is it like to imagine the future?

What is it like to imagine having HIV, or another STD?

What is personal commitment to HIV/STD prevention?

Why is HIV prevention important?

Content: Knowledge, Attitudes

Recommended Grade Level: 7-9

Correlation to Standards: Health Education: 1, 4, 6, 7; Science Education: E, F

Estimated Time: 15 minutes excluding Lesson Extension & Assessment

Part 1: Guided Imagery

1 Students close their eyes and relax into a comfortable position.

2 Students imagine themselves a year from now.

3 Ask what would students be doing if they had the freedom to be doing anything they wanted? What could give them a sense of happiness or satisfaction? With whom would they be — people they already know or people they hope to meet?

4 Students consider how they feel, now, as they imagine this scene from the future.

5 Students imagine going to get an HIV test just to make sure that they don't have HIV.

6 Students imagine how they would feel about waiting for the test results, especially because life is so good.

7 The test comes back positive. How would they feel? What changes would occur in their lives? Whom would they tell?

8 Students imagine, instead, that the test comes back negative. How would they feel? What changes would occur in their lives? Whom would they tell?

9 Change the scene from an HIV test to a test for one of the other STDs. Students imagine what it would be like to find out that they had herpes or gonorrhea or chlamydia rather than HIV.

10 Come back to the present. Students consider their own lives, now. What does each student need to do in order to prevent these diseases?

11 Ask students to make a silent, personal commitment — to themselves — to stay healthy.

12 After a minute of silence ask students to open their eyes and bring their attention back into the classroom when they are ready.

13 Discuss the experience of the guided imagery. What did the students think of the process?

- What will they walk away remembering?
- Was it helpful?

14 Reinforce the importance of preventing HIV, other STDs.

Lesson Extension & Assessment

1 Students write an essay or journal entry communicating the content of their personal commitment to stay safe (from Step 11, above).

2 Students use cartoon format to chart their course through the guided imagery section. Encourage students to use color and other artistic media to express their emotions. Display the cartoons. Alternatively, students choreograph a dance or compose music to express their reactions.

3 In small groups, students develop a guided imagery progression that would help promote prevention of high-risk behaviors such as the use of alcohol and other drugs.

4 Working individually, students identify media personalities whose lives have been impacted by HIV infection. Students write about the ways in which HIV has altered the course of these individual's lives.

Guiding Questions

What are ways to analyze the level of risk for HIV/STD transmission associated with different behaviors?

What is the level of risk of HIV/STD transmission associated with different behaviors?

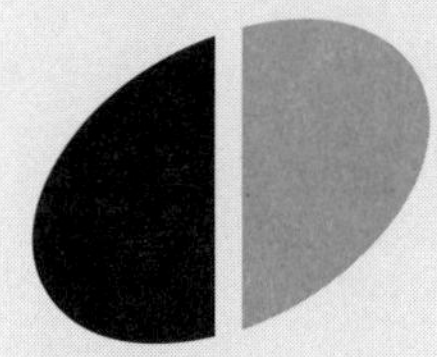

What are some developmentally appropriate risk reduction and risk elimination statements about HIV/STD prevention?

Content: Attitudes, Knowledge, Skills

Recommended Grade Level: 8-9

Correlation to Standards: Health Education: 1, 3, 5, 6, 7; Science Education: A, C, E, F, G

Estimated Time: 35 minutes excluding Lesson Extension & Assessment

Materials: One piece of paper and pen/pencil for each student.

Set Up: Create a space that is long enough for students to form a line standing shoulder to shoulder.

Part 1: The Risk Line

1. Distribute the scrap paper.
2. Ask the students to count off by threes (1, 2, 3) and write their number on the scrap paper.
3. Collect the pieces of paper, shuffle them and redistribute the scrap papers to the class with the numbers face down. Each student has a new number. Students should ignore the number they previously wrote down in step 2. (The reasoning behind the reassigning of numbers is so that students do not know each other's number.)
4. Draw the risk line on the board.

1	2	3
low-risk	some risk	high-risk

5. The numbers on the scrap paper correlate to the numbers on the risk line.
6. Students write a description of one hypothetical situation or behavior that

correlates to the number written on the scrap paper. For example, if the student has a "1," he/she should describe a low-risk situation or behavior.

7 Students imagine a risk line, similar to that drawn on the board, that stretches across the front of the classroom. Students silently place themselves on the imaginary line according to the riskiness of the behavior they described. Students do this part of the activity without communicating with each other.

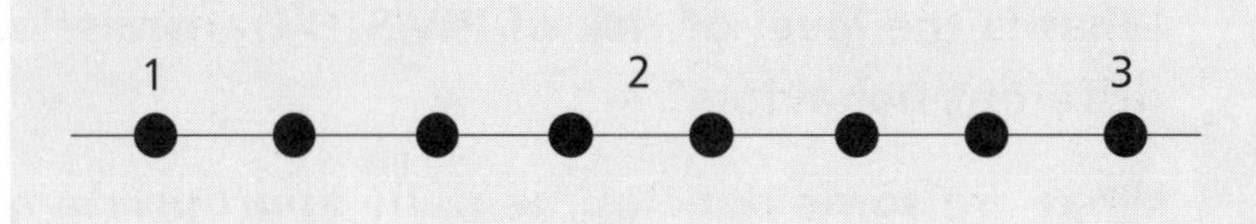

8 Once in line, each student describes the risk he/she represents.

The following behaviors should be included:

Low Risk — Abstinence from all behaviors with a risk of HIV/STD transmission; sexual intercourse in a trusting, mutually, monogamous relationship where both partners are HIV negative and have no other risky behaviors; kissing, holding hands etc.

Some Risk — Sexual intercourse with one partner (unknown HIV status) using a condom; sexual intercourse with multiple partners (unknown HIV status) using condoms.

High Risk — Unprotected oral-genital contact with one or more partners (unknown HIV status); unprotected sexual intercourse with one partner (unknown HIV status); unprotected sexual intercourse with multiple partners (unknown HIV status); sharing needles and other injection drug paraphernalia with a person(s) whose HIV status is unknown.

With less mature classes simply use the term sexual intercourse. With more mature classes, define sexual intercourse to include both vaginal and anal intercourse. If students have duplicate statements, reassign one of the students with a behavior that has not already been included.

NOTE: The term "low-risk" is used instead of "no risk" because students are often quick to point out that "it is possible, if unlikely, that something risky could happen."

9 Students rearrange themselves as needed to achieve the correct order on the line. Restate the risky behaviors to double check the sequence.

10 Beginning with the high-risk end of the line, each student presents a risk reduction strategy (safer) and a risk elimination strategy (safest) for his/her behavior. For low-risk behaviors, students present strategies to maintain the low-risk status.

11 Then, students move to the place on the line that reflects the application of their risk reduction strategy on the level of risk for the behavior they represent. They should only reduce their risk by one increment (i.e. unprotected intercourse -> condom use; or condom use -> abstinence).

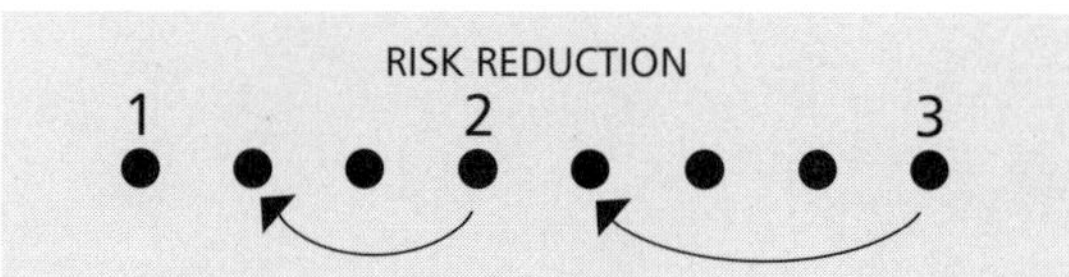

12 Discuss the risk reduction movement from high-risk to some risk, and some risk to low-risk. Discuss the fact that condom use involves some risk, not low-risk.

13 Discuss what would happen if everyone moved to the correct place in the line to reflect their risk elimination strategy. Ask the students to move to the place on the line that would reflect the application of a risk elimination strategy to the behavior they represent. Reinforce the importance of HIV prevention.

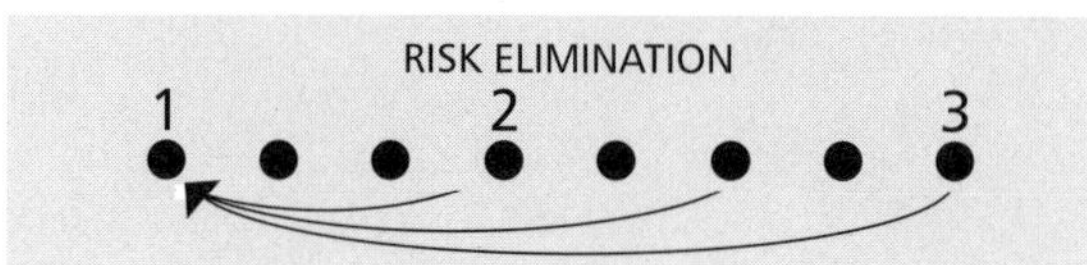

Lesson Extension & Assessment

1 Students draw the risk line on a piece of paper. Individually, students evaluate their own behaviors, and make a mark on the risk line to represent their current risk level. Students write responses to the questions below. Encourage students to regard their risk-lines as a contract with themselves to prevent HIV/STD infection.

- How can you reduce your own current risks or maintain a low-risk status?
- What factors might interfere with your ability to reduce your risks or maintain a low-risk status?
- What can you do to counter these factors so you can successfully reduce your risks or maintain a low-risk status?

2 In small groups, students apply the concepts from this activity to analyzing other types of risky behaviors such as substance use. Students develop and practice relevant risk elimination and risk reduction statements. Each group presents their analysis and statements to the class.

Guiding Questions

Does the media express attitudes or send messages about sex, sexuality and/or HIV/STDs?

What is a stereotype?

What is the role of critical thinking in evaluating media messages on sex, sexuality, and HIV/STDs?

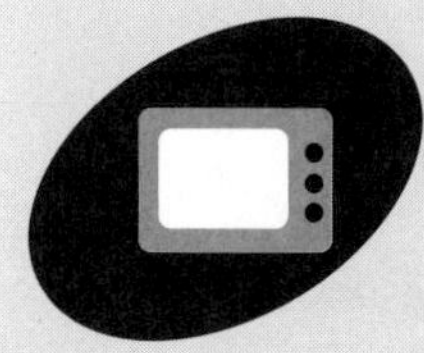

What are some developmentally appropriate alternative media messages for youth about sex, sexuality, and HIV/STDs?

Content: Attitudes, Skills

Recommended Grade Level: 7-9

Correlation to Standards: Health Education: 1, 4, 7; Science Education: A, F

Estimated Time: 35 minutes excluding Lesson Extension & Assessment

Materials: Various examples of magazines, newspapers, advertisements, radio clips, TV clips, online information, etc. that incorporate or reference sex, sexuality and/or HIV/STDs; poster paper and markers.

Part 1: The Media and Its Messages

1 What is the definition of the term *media*?

The term media refers to forms of mass communication that influence many people.

2 What are some examples of the media?

Radio, television, newspapers, and magazines.

3 What do the terms *sex* and **sexuality** mean?

Used loosely, the word "sex" can mean many things; it can refer to being male or female, the act of sexual intercourse, or sexual activity in general. Sexuality has to do with sexual character, a sense of sexual identity or sexual feelings.

4 What is a **stereotype**?

A stereotype is a simplified image or generalization that represents a thing or a group of people; often stereotypes are misleading and demeaning.

5 Students divide into small groups.

6. Each group takes a selection of the sample magazines, newspapers, advertisement, radio clips, TV clips, etc.
7. Groups review their samples and identify three media messages about sex, sexuality, and/or HIV/STDs.
8. Groups discuss and record short descriptions of these three messages.
9. Groups identify and record any stereotypes in the three examples.
10. Each group reports its findings to the class.

Part 2: Class Discussion

1. What kinds of messages does the media convey about sex? Is sex presented as cool or uncool?
2. Are there messages about eliminating and/or reducing the risk for HIV/STD infection? If so, what are the messages? If not, could there have been? What does the lack of attention to risk elimination and/or risk reduction tell us?
3. Are there media messages about sex, sexuality and HIV/STDs that are based on stereotypes? How about accurate information? How can a person tell the difference?
4. What does the media portray as being sexy? Are there different messages about sexiness for adults v. adolescents?
5. What do media messages communicate about peoples' appearance? Based on the media, what does the ideal male or female look like? Are these images realistic? Are they healthy? Do people buy into these images? If so, how?
6. What do media messages communicate about people with HIV, AIDS or other STDs?
7. Are there both **hidden** and **obvious** themes in the media about these topics? Which is more powerful? Why?
8. How can media messages about sex, sexuality, and HIV/STDs affect people's personal attitudes toward themselves? Toward others?
9. Can media messages affect people's behavior? If so, are people usually aware that the media has influenced their behavior? Why or why not?
10. Do media messages about sex, sexuality and HIV/STDs support a particular set of beliefs? If so, which ones? Whose perspectives are conveyed through the media?
11. How do the students feel about the kinds of messages they receive from the media regarding sex, sexuality and HIV/STDs?
12. Are there other messages that the students would like the media to present?

Lesson Extension & Assessment

1. Each group creates its own media messages regarding sex, sexuality and HIV/STDs. Each group writes the new messages for display on the poster paper. Groups present their messages to the class, and if possible, family or community members. Display the posters.
2. In small groups, students use art supplies to design images to match the messages developed in 1.
3. For homework, students write essays that critique movie, TV, or radio messages about sex, sexuality, or HIV/STDs.

Guiding Questions

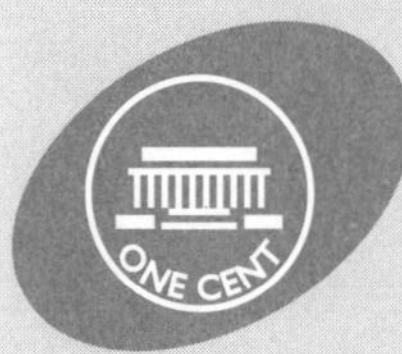

How does HIV attack the human immune system?

What are some of the challenges that scientists face in developing a cure for AIDS?

Is it possible to "see" who has HIV or AIDS?

Why is HIV prevention important for everybody?

Content: Knowledge, Attitudes

Recommended Grade Level: 5-9

Correlation to Standards: Health Education: 1, 2, 4, 7; Science Education: A, C, E, F, G

Estimated Time: 15 minutes excluding Lesson Extension & Assessment

Materials: Four pennies

Set Up: Create a large open space. (If time and/or space are limited, students can be seated during this activity.)

Part 1: Class Discussion

1 What is HIV?

2 What is the human immune system?

3 What are white blood cells?

4 Why is it important to have a healthy immune system?

Without a healthy immune system, a person could get very sick from many kinds of infections that would not otherwise be dangerous.

5 What are some examples of common infections that the human immune system can successfully fight off?

Examples include the flu, common cold, chicken pox etc.

6 Students move away from tables or desks and form a circle by standing shoulder to shoulder and facing inward.

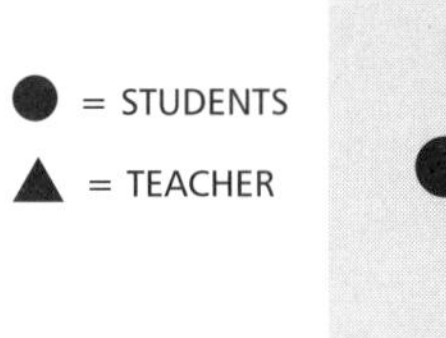

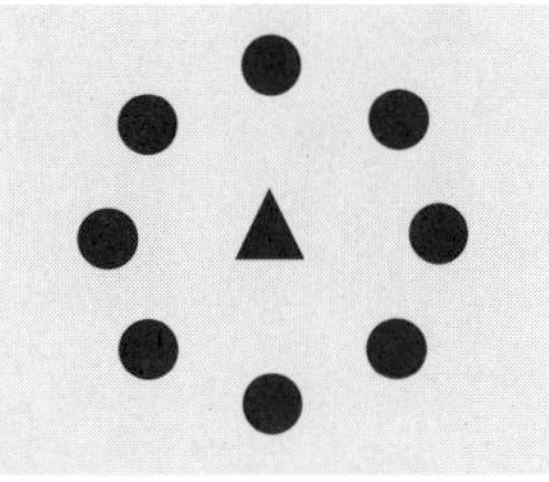

7 The teacher stands in the middle of the circle.

8 Mention that there are a few pennies in your hand which represent HIV. Students' hands represent white blood cells.

9 Students turn to face the outside of the circle so that their backs are towards you. Students put one hand out behind them (toward the center of the circle) with the palm facing up.

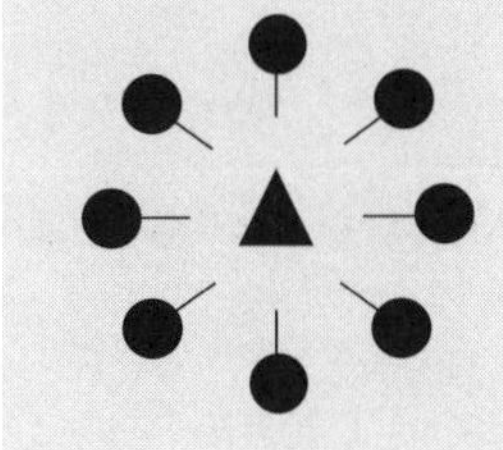

10 Walk around the inside of the circle and distribute the pennies into different students' hands.

11 Students close their hands (to make fists), whether or not they are holding pennies.

12 Students turn to face the inside of the circle.

13 Can the students tell which of the cells (fists) are infected with HIV (pennies) simply by looking at each other's hands?

No.

14 As a class, imagine that the students are scientists who are trying to find a way to get rid of the HIV inside a person's body.

15 How can the scientists see which cells are HIV infected?

They can "open up" the cells one by one.

16 What will "opening up" the cells do to the body?

"Opening up" the cells will kill both the HIV and the cells.

17 Demonstrate the process of "opening up the cells." Going around the circle, each student opens his/her fist one at a time.

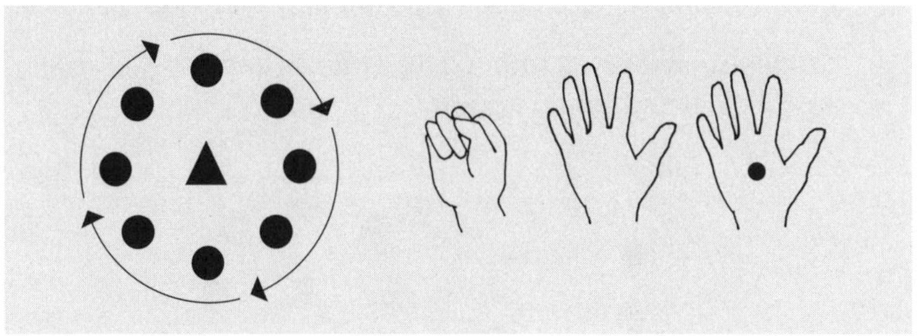

18 Should the class keep searching for more HIV in the circle after discovering the first penny?

Yes. There could be more hidden HIV (pennies).

19 Students continue opening their hands (killing healthy cells and HIV infected cells) until all of the pennies (viruses) are discovered and all the cells are dead.

20 What were the main points to this activity?

- HIV can hide inside human white blood **cells** just as the pennies could hide in the students' fists. Simply put, most substances that kill viruses in infected cells also kill healthy cells. There is still no cure for HIV.
- HIV hides inside an infected person's **body** in the same way that the virus hides inside white blood cells: HIV is not visible from the outside. You can not tell who has HIV by looking at a person's appearance.
- HIV can circulate freely in blood and infectious body fluids before entering cells, just like the teacher was able to hold the pennies and place them in students' hands.

21 Why is HIV prevention important for everybody?

Lesson Extension & Assessment

1 In small groups, students brainstorm possible ideas about getting HIV out of the body without killing all the cells. Then, students research different strategies that today's scientists are currently exploring to treat HIV infection and AIDS. Groups present their research to the class.

2 Students repeat the Pennies Activity at home with their families and write up their experiences teaching about HIV prevention.

3 In small groups, students consider the difference between private information and public information. What do people learn about each other through casual experience? What are the kinds of things that are kept personal? How does this relate to health? Do people have the right to know if someone has an infectious disease that is transmitted through casual contact, such as by a sneeze or cough? How about a disease like HIV that is transmitted in very specific ways that are not casual? Groups create suggested guidelines for what kind of health information could be public v. private. Each group presents its guidelines to the class.

Guiding Questions

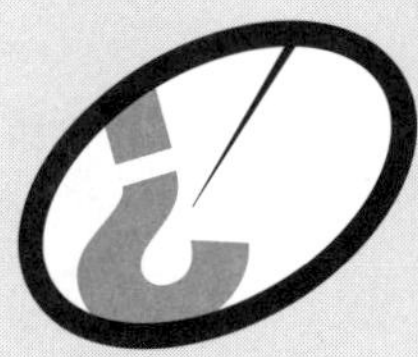

What is the HIV antibody test?

What is the role of the three month window period in the HIV antibody test?

What are some of the reasons people get an HIV antibody test?

Why is HIV prevention important?

Content: Attitudes, Knowledge

Recommended Grade Level: 7-9

Correlation to Standards: Health Education 1, 2, 3, 5, 7; Science Education: A, C, E, F, G

Estimated Time: 15 minutes excluding Lesson Extension & Assessment

---

Part 1: Review of HIV Antibody Test Information

1 See the chapter entitled Information About HIV and AIDS.

Part 2: The Test

1 Discuss the differences between analogies and facts. Note that this activity uses an analogy to explain the HIV antibody test. Emphasize that the imaginary purple dye discussed in this activity is not HIV. HIV does not make a person turn purple.

2 Recruit two student volunteers.

3 Explain that you have an imaginary, sterile hypodermic needle in each of your hands. Both needles contain purple liquids. One of the liquids is a harmless purple dye that, once injected, will cause a person's skin to turn purple three months later. The other purple liquid is also harmless but it does not cause the person's skin to change color.

4 Pretend to inject each student volunteer with one of the purple fluids. Do not indicate which needle contains the purple dye.

5 Explain that the only way to know which student received the dye is to conduct a visual test three months later. After three months, the skin of the person with the dye will turn purple.

Part 3: Class Discussion

1 Can anyone tell immediately which student was injected with the dye?

No, the visual test is only accurate when applied three months after the injection since the dye does not color the skin until then.

2 Imagine that two months have passed. Is it now possible to tell who received dye?

No.

3 State that the full three months have passed. Identify the student who received the injection of purple dye. Ask the class to imagine that this student's skin is bright purple

4 How long was the purple dye inside the "purple" student?

Three months.

5 What are the similarities between the purple dye and its visual test and HIV and the HIV antibody test?

- This activity uses an analogy: the purple dye is like HIV and the visual test for purple dye is like the HIV test.
- Both tests require a three month waiting period for accurate results.
- Three months after injection of the purple dye/HIV infection, it is possible to detect the body's reaction to the dye/virus.
- Both tests measure the body's reaction to the dye or virus, rather than detecting the dye or the virus themselves.

6 Are there any differences between the purple dye and its visual test and HIV and the HIV antibody test?

- The test for the dye is a visual test, meaning that everyone who can see the person three months after the last possible dye injection can tell if he/she received the dye.
- The HIV test is a blood test. The antibodies are not visible to the naked eye. People with HIV infection do not look different from people who are uninfected.

7 What would have happened if two purple injections were given to the same student — the first in January (harmless fluid) and the second, in February (purple dye)? Would a visual test be accurate in March? Why? When should the student have a test in order to obtain an accurate result? Compare to HIV testing.

No, the test is accurate three months after the last time the dye could have been introduced into a person's body. In this case, the person could have received the dye in January as well as February. A test done in March could determine whether the student received the dye in January, but this test will not give an accurate indication about the February injection.

The student should wait until a full three months have passed from the last possible time the dye could have been introduced into his/her body.

8 Do people with HIV turn purple?

No. The purple dye discussed in this activity is purely imaginary and has no real relationship to HIV.

9 Is it possible to know the exact number of people in one's community, country, or the world that become infected with HIV? Can we know how many people will actually take the HIV antibody test?

10 Does a negative HIV antibody test result guarantee that a person will never get HIV?

No, the only way to avoid HIV is for a person to make safe(r) choices about his or her behavior. **Prevention works.**

1 Individually, students complete the following tasks:

Imagine that you are talking to a friend about his/her behavior and risk of HIV infection. Based on your understanding of HIV transmission and prevention, you think that your friend might have been exposed to HIV. Write your responses to the following questions:

- Would you suggest that your friend get an HIV test?
- Why/why not?
- What would you say?
- How do you think he/she might respond?
- How do you think you would feel about this discussion?
- How do you think your friend would feel?
- What other HIV-related issues could you talk about with your friend?

2 In small groups, students develop skits based on the responses to the questions above. Groups present their skits to the class, and invite family and community members to attend.

3 Individually or in small groups, students create analogies (other than the purple dye) for explaining the role of antibodies and the three month window period in HIV testing. Students showcase their analogies in written text and/or verbal presentations.

4 Individually or in small groups, students interview medical professionals and document the proper procedures for drawing blood and giving injections. Students design a creative, visual format through which to present a step-by-step narrative for these procedures. Encourage students to begin their documentation with the preparation of the needles and conclude with what happens to the used needle, donated blood, and/or empty containers holding whatever was injected. Display the narratives for the school community.

5 Individually, students write essays presenting their responses to the question, "Is it good public health policy to make everyone in the United States have an HIV test once a year?" Students should consider issues of civil rights, the cost of tests v. the cost of not testing, what message(s) such a policy might send, the implications of the window period, and other potential benefits as well as costs to the U.S. Alternately, conduct a class debate on the issue of mandatory HIV testing.

Guiding Questions

How does the model of a "decision-making chain" represent connections between choices and decisions that can lead to risk-taking behaviors?

Can the "decision-making chain" model be used to evaluate the risks of HIV/STD infection?

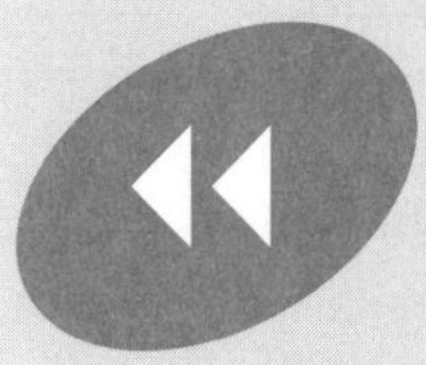

What are some HIV/STD prevention risk reduction and risk elimination statements appropriate for specific hypothetical scenarios?

Content: Attitudes, Skills

Recommended Grade Level: 8-9

Correlation to Standards: Health Education: 1, 3, 6; Science Education: A, F

Estimated Time: 35 minutes excluding Lesson Extension & Assessment

Part 1: Activity

1. Students divide into working groups of approximately five people.

2. Each group identifies a behavior that has a high-risk for HIV/STD infection. Working backwards in terms of time chronology, each group identifies the critical decisions that lead to the high-risk behavior. The groups should identify as many steps, inclusive of the outcome, as there are people in the group (5 people = 5 steps).

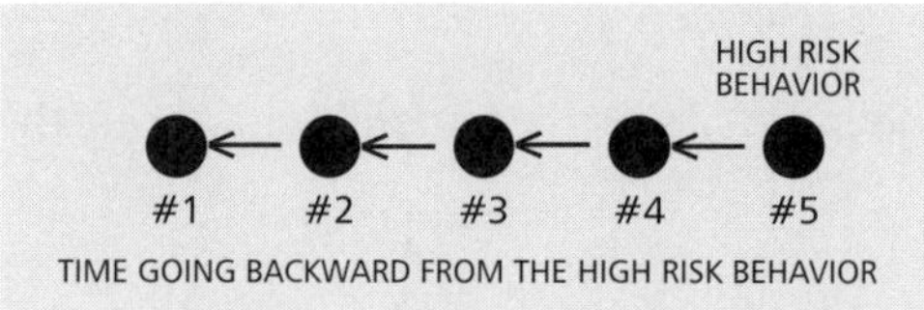

For example, unprotected intercourse is a high-risk behavior (#5) that resulted from going alone into a bedroom with another person (#4) after drinking too much and getting drunk (#3) at a big, unsupervised party (#2) to which the person went without a condom (#1).

NOTE: If all the groups are using the same outcome, suggest that some groups choose a different topic.

3. After identifying and choosing the steps, each group identifies other available options for each decision-making juncture.

For example, with regard to alcohol, what options does a person have (not drinking, drinking but not getting drunk, getting drunk in a situation where sex is likely, getting drunk in a situation where sex is unlikely, etc.)?

4 Examine which option(s) could have changed the course of the risk-taking progression either by reducing or eliminating the risk of HIV/STD infection. In other words, *what could have happened if the person who had unprotected intercourse when drunk had decided not to drink...*

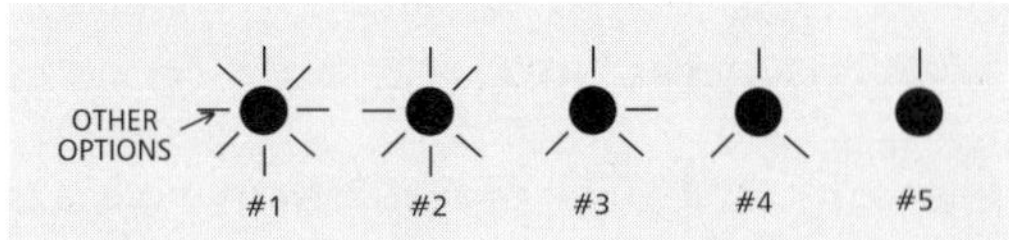

5 Each group forms a line (in chronological sequence by step) and practices presenting the progression of the decisions leading to the high-risk behavioral outcome. Then, each person in the line steps forward to present the risk reduction and the risk elimination options for his or her specific step.

6 Groups present their decision-making chains, step by step, to the class.

Part 2: Class Discussion

1 What is the "decision-making chain?" Why did we do this activity? Was the visual presentation helpful in understanding the progression of risk-taking decisions?

2 Why did the groups present risk reduction as well as risk elimination options? Discuss the chain reaction in the decision-making progression, i.e. how does the first step toward risky behavior effect the ultimate outcome?

3 Who is responsible for the risk-taking process? Do people usually have control over their risks? What are some situations in which an individual has no control? What can be done about these kinds of situations?

4 How hard is it to talk about concerns involved with risk-taking? What can be at stake if a person expresses doubts about taking risks that his/her peers are in favor of?

5 What can help people be more confident about their ability to control their own risks?

6 When is a good time to think about preventing a high-risk behavior?

7 Review the connections between substance use and high-risk sexual behavior. Discuss transmission routes including needle sharing, as well as sexual behavior and physical violence under the influence of alcohol and/or other drugs.

8 What, if any, types of high-risk behaviors were not explored by any of the groups? Verbally apply the progression of this activity to evaluating previously unexamined scenarios.

9 How could students adapt the progression of this activity to be useful in their own risk-taking decisions?

10 Reinforce the importance of preventing HIV infection and other STDs.

Lesson Extension & Assessment

1 Apply the decision-making chain to risky behaviors other than those that can lead to HIV/STD transmission. Apply the decision-making chain to healthy behaviors. Compare and contrast.

2 Working individually, students practice self observation by noticing and recording their decision-making processes and outcomes for a set period of time. How many decisions did the students make quickly and easily; how many decisions were harder, requiring more thought? Did students use a decision-making chain? If so, students chart the process. If not, how did students make decisions? What did students learn from this exercise?

Guiding Questions

What are the different HIV/STD transmission risks associated with teens' behaviors at parties?

What are the health benefits of low-risk behaviors at parties?

What kinds of parties promote high-risk behaviors? Low risk behaviors?

What are appropriate risk reduction and risk elimination strategies for promoting safety at parties?

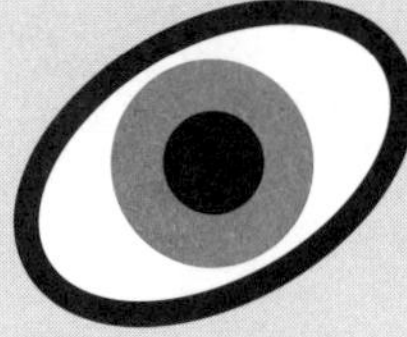

Are there connections between critical thinking skills and the communication skills helpful in risk elimination and risk reduction?

Content: Attitudes, Skills

Recommended Grade Level: 8-9

Correlation to Standards: Health Education: 1, 3, 4, 5, 6, 7; Science Education: A, F

Estimated Time: 35 minutes excluding Lesson Extension & Assessment

Materials: One piece of paper and pen/pencil for each student.

Part 1: The Risk of a Party

1. Ask students about the social changes they expect during the next year. For example, will they have more freedom? More work? Will their social life change? Lead into a discussion on parties.

2. Draw the risk line on the board.

Parties	
low-risk	high-risk

NOTE: The term "low-risk" is used instead of "no risk" because students are often quick to point out that "it is possible, if unlikely, that something risky could happen."

3. Students divide into two groups. One group thinks of a party scenario that would promote behaviors with a high risk of HIV/STD transmission. The group lists

some possible characteristics of this party under the appropriate heading on the board.

4 The other group thinks of a party scenario that would promote behavior with a low-risk of HIV/STD transmission. This group lists some of the possible characteristics of a low-risk party under the appropriate heading on the board.

Possible characteristics can include: the size of the party; the ages of the people present; degree of adult supervision; availability of drugs and alcohol; the sex of the people present; the likelihood of violence; the location; etc.

5 As a class, discuss strategies to reduce the risk of behaviors associated with HIV/STD transmission for each high-risk characteristic.

For example, if party size is a variable, then a large party is more likely to permit/foster high-risk behaviors. Risk reduction strategies for attending a large party can include:

- going to the party with a small group of friends and staying with them at the party,
- staying in public areas while at the party,
- including friends in socializing with "new people", etc.

6 Draw an arrow (←) pointing from high-risk toward low-risk to demonstrate the degree of risk reduction achieved with each strategy.

7 Draw a star (★) by each low-risk behavior and reinforce the positive health benefits associated with behaviors that have a low-risk of HIV/STD transmission.

8 How do the characteristics of the low-risk party contribute to low-risk behaviors?

9 What are some strategies that reinforce and support low-risk behaviors (i.e. spending time with friends who have similar risk tolerances and who support low-risk behaviors).

10 Do any of the characteristics associated with parties that foster behaviors with a high-risk of HIV/STD transmission also contribute to other high-risk behaviors (i.e. can the presence of alcohol contribute to the risk of violent behavior?).

11 What is the risk of unintended pregnancy associated with some behaviors that also have a risk of HIV/STD transmission?

12 Ask students if the progression outlined in this activity was useful. Could this progression be useful in future situations?

13 Are all "cool" parties automatically high-risk? Can low-risk parties be fun?

14 How can students control their own level of risk of HIV/STD transmission?

Part 2: Written Follow-Up

1 Working individually, students draw a risk line.

2 Students consider their own current risk level for HIV/STD transmission and write "now" on the appropriate point on the risk line.

3 Students imagine their risk levels for next year and write "next year" on the appropriate point on the risk line.

4 Students write responses to the following questions:

- How can you reduce your own current risks or maintain your low-risk status?
- What can you do to reduce your projected risks or maintain your low-risk status?
- What factors might interfere with your ability to reduce your risks or maintain your low-risk status?
- What can you do to counter these factors so you can successfully reduce your risks or maintain your low-risk status?

5 Revisit the progression of identifying risk, formulating risk elimination/risk reduction strategies, and using the strategies successfully.

Lesson Extension and Assessment

1 In small groups, students evaluate other relevant social situations for risk related to HIV/STD infection. Students apply the concepts for this activity to their analysis. Each group presents its findings to the class, and family members, if possible.

2 Working individually, students address the tension between the factors that promote high-risk behaviors and reasons for avoiding these same high-risk behaviors. Why are some high-risk behaviors so compelling? Do some people consciously decide to avoid these behaviors? How much control does an individual have in his/her own life? What is the role of life experience in building confidence and staying safe? What can help people learn important lessons about prevention without endangering themselves? Do students have helpful suggestions on this topic for youth in lower grades?

Guiding Questions

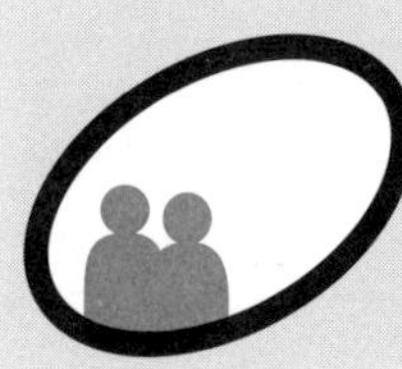

What are some possible health effects of STDs and pregnancy?

What is the relationship between STDs, pregnancy and the risk of HIV infection?

How do the issues of personal responsibility, consequences and stereotypes relate to HIV, STDs, and pregnancy?

What are developmentally appropriate risk elimination and risk reduction statements about HIV, STD, and pregnancy?

Content: Attitudes, Knowledge, Skills

Recommended Grade Level: 7-9

Correlation to Standards: Health Education 1, 2, 4, 6, 7; Science Education: A, C, E, F, G

Estimated Time: 35 minutes excluding Lesson Extension & Assessment

Materials: Research Handout; poster paper and markers.

Part 1: Information on STDs & Pregnancy

1. Brainstorm as a class to list the names of common STDs. Include slang names as appropriate, i.e. "the clap" for gonorrhea. Also, list pregnancy on the blackboard, but make it clear that pregnancy is NOT a STD.

   The final list should include chancroid, chlamydia, genital herpes, genital warts (human papoloma virus), gonorrhea, granuloma inguinale, hepatitis B, HIV, pubic lice (crabs) and scabies, syphilis, and trichomoniasis. (HIV is not covered here due to the in-depth coverage provided throughout the manual)

2. Students divide into small groups.

3. Assign the topic of one or more STDs from the list on the board to each group for research purposes.

4. Each group researches its assigned STD or pregnancy and creates a poster that communicates the answers to the research questions. Groups can use the library, internet, community resources etc. for research purposes. Groups display their posters.

   (see next page for research questions)

For STDs:

1 What causes this disease?

2 What are the symptoms of this disease?

3 How is this disease transmitted?

4 Is this disease curable?

5 Is this disease treatable?

6 Does this disease pose specific problems for pregnant women and their fetuses/babies?

7 Does this disease increase the risk of HIV infection? If so, how?

8 How can this disease be prevented?

For Pregnancy:

1 What causes a pregnancy?

2 How does a female know she is pregnant?

3 What are a woman's options regarding her pregnancy?

4 How can pregnancy be prevented?

5 Students read the information on the other groups' posters. Each group is considered an expert resource on its topic. In large class format, students ask and answer questions about the different research topics and information displayed on the posters.

Part 2: Risk Elimination and Risk Reduction

1 Groups reconvene and address issues of responsibility, consequences, and stereotypes pertaining to the selected topic(s). Groups consider their assigned topic(s) and list their responses to the following questions to use later for a class presentation:

- Whom does this condition affect — directly and/or indirectly?
- What are the responsibilities of the person who has this condition?
- What are the potential consequences of this condition? For whom? When?
- What are the stereotypes associated with this condition?

2 Each group presents the responses to the entire class.

3 Discuss the students' responses to the questions listed above. In particular, challenge stereotypes.

Sample discussion topics include the following questions:

- Consider two sexually active people, one of whom has a sexually transmitted disease. Why do many people think the person with the disease is somehow dirtier than the other person who didn't get a STD? Remember, they were both taking the same risk.
- Is there a difference in the way people view a sexually active male and a sexually active female? What about if the male and female have multiple sexual partners? What are the words often used to describe males and females in these situations? Why are men with HIV still assumed to be homosexual?
- Why are STDs viewed differently than any other type of communicable disease?
- Are there differences between disease prevention and pregnancy prevention? If yes, what are they? If no, why not?

  The justification for disease prevention is fairly straightforward — people usually want to avoid disease. In contrast, pregnancy may be desirable or undesirable depending on personal circumstances.

  In addition, there are many forms of birth control that can help HIV/STD infection.

- Are there similarities between disease prevention and pregnancy prevention? If yes, what are they? If no, why not?

Both can be prevented through risk elimination and risk reduction.

- Are there similarities between risk elimination and risk reduction? If yes, what are they? If no, why not?

  Both can require an active choice that supports prevention.

- Are there differences between risk elimination and risk reduction? If yes, what are they? If no, why not?

  Unlike risk reduction, risk elimination is 100% safe.

Lesson Extension & Assessment

1 In their small groups, students develop and implement an assessment tool to measure the educational outcomes of the presentations on STDs and pregnancy. In other words, what kinds of activities could allow students to demonstrate how well they learned the information and concepts presented in these activities?

2 Each student uses the posters as resources from which to write a review of the main points about each of the STDs and pregnancy.

3 Students individually rank the STDs and pregnancy in order of their consequences — most severe to least severe. Students write short speeches that explain the ranking order. Students present their speeches to the entire class. With the teacher's assistance, the class reaches a decision on ranking by consensus.

NOTE: There are many acceptable ranking orders for this task. Students should be able to justify their choices.

4 Working individually, each student considers what he/she could say to a sexual partner to insist upon risk elimination as well as risk reduction. Would he/she mention disease prevention? Pregnancy prevention (when appropriate)? Would he/she justify the choice or simply state it? Students write their responses or turn to the people next to them and exchange

Guiding Questions

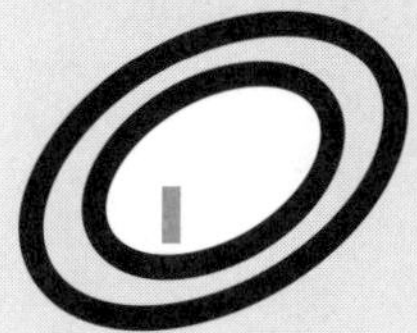

What is a condom?

What are the health benefits of condom use?

What is risk elimination?

What is risk reduction?

Content: Attitudes, Skills, Knowledge

Recommended Grade Level: 5-6

Correlation to Standards: Health Education: 1, 3; Science Education: A, C, E, F, G

Estimated Time: 10 minutes excluding Lesson Extension & Assessment

Part 1: Class Discussion

1 What is a condom?

A condom is a barrier that is similar to a glove. A condom covers a man's penis as a glove covers a hand. Condoms are usually made out of thin rubber or rubber-like substances.

2 Why do people use condoms?

People use condoms to help prevent the spread of HIV and other STDs during sexual intercourse and/or to help prevent pregnancy. However, condoms can break or leak and cannot guarantee safety from HIV/STD infection or pregnancy.

3 Can condoms make sex completely safe?

No. Condoms can prevent HIV, STDs, and pregnancy. However, condoms cannot make sex 100% safe. The only sure way not to get HIV, STDs or have an unintended pregnancy is not to have sex.

4 Can condoms reduce the risk of HIV, other STDs, and pregnancy?

Yes, using condoms can reduce the risk of HIV, STDs and pregnancy. Using condoms is a risk reduction strategy.

5 How can a person avoid the risk of HIV, other STDs or unintended pregnancy

From a health perspective, the only certain way to be totally safe from HIV, STDs, and unintended pregnancy is not to have sex, share needles, or do anything that poses a risk of infection. Abstaining from sex is a risk elimination strategy. It is safest to wait and have sex only when you are in a long-term, trusting relationship where both people are disease-free and have no other risks.

6 Do people need to use condoms forever?

From a health perspective, people do not need to use condoms to prevent HIV/STD transmission when they are in a very serious, committed, trusting, risk-free relationship where both people know they are healthy because each person has had a test for HIV. (People may still choose to use condoms to reduce the risk of a pregnancy.)

7 What should you do if you find a (used) condom on the street?

It is best not to touch things you find in the street whether they are condoms or other unfamiliar objects. Find an adult and tell him/her that you found a condom (or something unfamiliar) and show the adult where it it is.

Suggest that the adult use plastic bags or housecleaning gloves to move the condom. The condom, along with anything that touched the condom, should be thrown away in a plastic garbage bag.

Lesson Extension & Assessment

1 Working individually, students write their own responses to the questions outlined above. Check for accuracy.

Guiding Questions

What are the limitations and benefits of correct and consistent condom use?

What are the positive health benefits of risk elimination regarding HIV/STD prevention?

What are the positive health benefits of risk reduction regarding HIV/STD prevention?

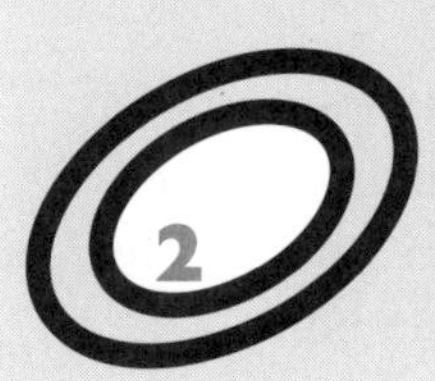

What are some developmentally appropriate risk elimination and risk reduction statements?

Content: Attitudes, Skills

Recommended Grade Level: 7-9

Correlation to Standards: Health Education: 1, 3, 5, 6, 7; Science Education: A, C, E, F, G

Estimated Time: 15 minutes excluding Lesson Extension & Assessment

Materials: One condom for the teacher's use only.

Part 1: Class Discussion

1 What does the word *sex* mean?

Sex often means sexual intercourse (oral, vaginal or anal).

2 Are people at risk for HIV/STD infection when they have sex?

Vaginal intercourse poses a risk of HIV/STD infection. Oral and anal intercourse present a risk for HIV/STD infection.

3 What does risk elimination mean?

The practice of avoiding all risks of HIV/STD infection is called risk elimination.

4 What does risk reduction mean?

The practice of using condoms to help prevent HIV/STD infection is called risk reduction.

5 What are condoms designed to do?

Condoms are designed to prevent the exchange of sexual fluids, including semen, pre-ejaculatory fluid, vaginal secretions and blood. When used correctly and consistently latex or polyurethane condoms can prevent HIV/STD infection.

NOTE: Condoms can only help prevent those infections transmitted through fluids or skin contact that are covered by the condom. A STD located outside the area covered by the condom will still be very infectious.

6 What kinds of condoms can be effective?

Latex or polyurethane condoms used with spermicidal lubricant or plain, water-based lubricant can prevent HIV/STD infection.

7 Where is it best to store condoms?

Condoms are sensitive to cold, heat, friction, and pressure. Besides cabinets or drawers, it is best to store condoms in front pockets, purses, packs, or other relatively cool protected places. Never store condoms in wallets, cars or other places where the condom or condom packaging could be damaged.

8 Does the correct and consistent use of condoms guarantee HIV/STD prevention?

No. The only certain way to prevent HIV/STD infection is not to do anything risky.

9 So, why do people use condoms at all?

Condoms can prevent HIV/ and many other STDs, even though they are not 100% safe. Condoms can make sex less dangerous for people who choose to take the risk of having sexual intercourse before they are able to have safe sex.

General information:

Condoms do not guarantee HIV/STD prevention. Condoms can fail. For example, they can break if air is trapped in the tip of the condom during use; there can be small tears from handling, etc.

Correct and consistent use of condoms typically requires a high degree of responsibility and commitment on the part of sexual partners. While a small number of condoms fail because they are defective, the vast majority of condom failures result from incorrect and inconsistent **use**.

Water-based lubricants can be used with condoms to reduce the chance of condom failure from friction and dryness. However, petroleum-based lubricants can damage latex condoms and should not be used.

Both sexual partners are responsible for the use of protection, since both partners make the choice to take the risk of having sex.

Condoms do not provide any protection from diseases that affect body parts not covered by the condom, such as a herpes sore on the outside of the vagina or on any exposed areas of a man's genitals.

Part 2: Condom Demonstration

1 Conduct the following demonstration with a lubricated latex or polyurethane condom. Explain and demonstrate the steps for correct condom use by unrolling the condom on the extended middle and index fingers of one hand to represent an erect penis. Keep the demonstration brief.

Before Ejaculation:

- Always use a new condom and check for expiration date.
- Check the packaging of the condom for rips or tears. Is the condom surrounded by an intact air pocket?
- Push the condom away from one corner of the packaging and carefully tear the package open from that corner without ripping the condom.
- Remove the condom from the packaging by pushing on the wrapper at the base of the condom and gently moving the condom out.
- Condoms must be put on before any genital contact occurs, since vaginal secretions, pre-ejaculatory fluid, and semen can transmit HIV and other STDs.
- Condoms only unroll in one direction. Determine which way the condom unrolls by using the fingers to unroll the condom slightly before attempting to unroll the condom onto the penis. Do not use a condom that has been put onto the penis inside-out since the pre-ejaculatory fluid on the tip of the penis may contaminate the condom.
- Unroll the condom about one inch onto an erect penis (fingers).
- Squeeze the air out of the condom to leave room for the semen at the tip of the condom.
- Roll the condom completely down to the base of the penis (as represented by the knuckles).

After Ejaculation:

- Hold onto the condom at the base of the penis (fingers) so that the condom does not fall off during withdrawal. The penis should be withdrawn immediately after ejaculation to help prevent condom leakage that could occur as the penis becomes smaller and softer.
- The condom should be taken off carefully, with the tip pointing down, to avoid spilling the semen.

Lesson Extension & Assessment

1 In small groups, students brainstorm responses to the questions listed below. Groups summarize and present their responses to the class.

- What is the role of communication between sexual partners in correct and consistent use of condoms?
- Who is responsible for using condoms?
- When does the responsibility for using condoms begin?
- What might interfere with a person's commitment and ability to use condoms?
- What might strengthen a person's commitment and ability to use condoms?
- What is the difference between risk reduction and risk elimination? Why is risk elimination the safest choice?

2 In small groups, students develop, practice and present risk elimination and risk reduction statements in response to the arguments listed below.

- "Condoms are a pain. I don't want to use them."
- "We haven't been using condoms so why should we start now? I mean, either we've already got HIV or we're not going to get it."

  NOTE: People can be infected with HIV with only one exposure. It is also possible to be exposed to HIV and not be infected, but this does not guarantee that infection will not occur the next time. Therefore, couples should make the commitment to use condoms even if they have not in the past. In addition, if two HIV-infected people have unprotected sex, they can become re-infected with each other's different HIV mutations.

- "I only use condoms with people I don't know well."
- "Condoms are a turn off."
- "I don't know where or how to get condoms. Also, I'd be really embarrassed to buy them — what if someone saw me?"
- "There's gonna be a cure for AIDS soon, so it doesn't matter if I get HIV now."

3 Invite family members to create support statements that affirm the students' statements by reinforcing the message of risk elimination (and risk reduction).

4 As an essay assignment or journal entry, students explore the reasoning behind their personal risk elimination and risk reduction statements. Are students optimistic about their ability to communicate these statements successfully in real-life situations? What might stand in their way? How can they increase their chances of being safe?

5 As an essay assignment or journal entry, students write and sign a personal pledge regarding risk elimination or risk reduction. Students save their pledge in portfolios.

6 In small groups, students design their own class progression to cover the same content included in this activity.

Guiding Questions

What is risk elimination? Risk reduction?

What is verbal communication? Non-verbal communication?

What is the role of assertive verbal and non-verbal communication in HIV/STD prevention?

What are some developmentally appropriate verbal and non-verbal strategies to eliminate the risk of HIV/STDs?

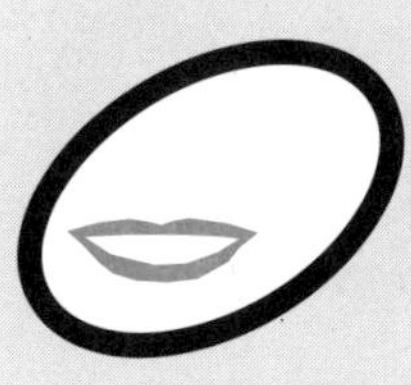

What are some developmentally appropriate verbal and non-verbal strategies to reduce the risk of HIV/STDs?

Content: Attitudes/Perceptions, Skills

Recommended Grade Level: 7-9

Correlation to Standards: Health Education: 1, 3, 4, 5, 6, 7; Science Education: A, F

Time Estimate: 35 minutes excluding Lesson Extension & Assessment

Materials: Poster papers and markers.

Part 1: Class Discussion

1 What is verbal communication?

Talking about something.

2 What is non-verbal communication?

Expressing something without using spoken words; this might involve body language,etc.

3 What are some examples of verbal and non-verbal communication that are common to everyone's experience?

4 What is risk elimination?

The practice of avoiding all risks of HIV/STDs infection is called risk elimination.

5 What is risk reduction?

The practice of using condoms to help prevent HIV/ STD infection is called risk reduction.

Part 2: Activity

1. Students divide into small groups.
2. Groups pick one hypothetical sexual behavior and one non-sexual behavior that have a high-risk of HIV/STD infection.
3. Groups brainstorm on how people can talk about HIV /STD prevention before engaging in the hypothetical high-risk behaviors.

   For example:

   - Two people involved romantically can talk about their desire to wait to have sex until they are older.
   - People can talk about using condoms before having sex.
   - A client in a tattoo parlor can request information regarding the tattoo parlor's disease prevention procedures prior to getting a tattoo.
4. Each student in every group develops and shares **one verbal** and **one non-verbal risk elimination** and **risk reduction** statement per scenario.
5. Each group selects the strongest verbal and non-verbal risk elimination and risk reduction statements, writes the statements on the poster paper, and presents them to the class.

Part 3: Class Discussion

1. Are there common themes or messages among the verbal risk elimination statements?
2. Do the statements from the groups sound similar or different — consider tone, length and word choice? Why or why not? What about the verbal risk reduction statements?

   Usually, there are more similarities than differences; the statements are clear, short, assertive.
3. Are there common characteristics or qualities to the non-verbal risk elimination statements? The non-verbal risk reduction statements?
4. Are the verbal and non-verbal risk reduction and risk elimination statements useful and/or usable? Why or why not?
5. Would using a combination of verbal and non-verbal statements be more successful than using just one or the other?
6. Would it be more effective to use a verbal or a non-verbal statement first? Why?
7. What type of statement — verbal or non-verbal — do people tend to make when they feel confident and in control? How about when people feel threatened or insecure? Which kinds of statements seem easier to make? Why?
8. Compare and contrast the following terms: *aggressive* and *assertive*. Are

aggressive risk elimination and/or risk reduction statements likely to be more effective than assertive statements? Why or why not?

NOTE: **Assertive** statements are usually more effective. **Aggressive** statements can be threatening and lead to anger; assertive statements tend to be confident and less likely to escalate tension. (The teacher can model an assertive and aggressive statement for the class if needed.)

9 What can help people feel confident about making verbal and/or non-verbal risk elimination or risk reduction statements? What can make it harder for people to make these types of statements?

10 When is the best time to define your risk elimination or risk reduction position — before or after entering a potentially high-risk situation?

Lesson Extension & Assessment

1 Working individually, students write descriptions of two risky behaviors that they might be confronted with in the (near) future. Students then develop and describe assertive, verbal and non-verbal **risk elimination** and **risk reduction** statements appropriate for each of their identified risky behaviors.

2 Students use cartoon images to communicate their verbal and non-verbal risk elimination and risk reduction statements. Display the artwork.

3 Discuss the issues of physical and emotional safety related to a person's ability to communicate about HIV/ STDs. See the Emotional and Physical Safety Discussion. Students write essays or journal entries about the connections, or lack thereof between emotional/physical safety and risk elimination/risk reduction.

4 Students watch a designated TV show/movie and record the verbal/non-verbal statements made by the main characters. Students develop and present a TV/movie review focusing on the communication strategies used during the show.

"Walk Like" Activity

Guiding Questions

What is a stereotype? Can stereotypes affect how people respond to people with HIV or AIDS?

What is discrimination? Is discrimination a relevant concern for people with HIV or AIDS?

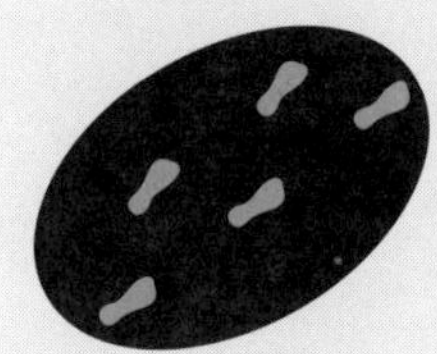

What do students think about people with HIV or AIDS? What is it like to imagine having HIV or AIDS?

Why is HIV prevention important?

Content: Attitudes

Recommended Grade Level: 5-9

Correlation to Standards: Health Education: 1, 4, 7; Science Education: F, G

Estimated Time: 15 minutes excluding Lesson Extension & Assessment

Set Up: Create an open space in which students can walk freely.

Part 1: Walking Toward Empathy

1 Guide students to walk in different ways, showing specific characteristics, according to the teacher's directions listed below. Students express a variety of emotions and physical conditions in sequence by changing the manner in which they walk. Regardless of their specific task, students walk silently throughout the activity. Direct students to:

- Walk normally.
- Walk like you have sprained ankles.
- Walk like you're proud of yourselves.
- Walk like you're tired.
- Walk like you're feeling really good.
- Walk like you're very sad.
- Walk like you're confused.
- Walk like you're comfortable with yourselves and know exactly where you're going.
- Walk like you have AIDS or HIV.

Part 2: Class Discussion

1 Did students adopt similar or dissimilar body language to each other during the previous steps ?

Most likely, people walked similarly during each step.

2 Was the response to the last step, "walk like you have AIDS or HIV."?

In almost all cases, at least one student walks "normally." Others typically stop, stare at each other, look confused at the teacher, or shrug their shoulders.

3 Did students limp when asked to walk like they had a sprained ankle?

Most likely, yes.

4 If so, does the entire class currently have sprained ankles?

Probably not.

5 If not, why did everyone limp?

Most people have had a sprained ankle or seen someone who has.

6 Can someone who does not have HIV (or does not know if he/she has HIV) nonetheless try to imagine what it might be like to be infected with HIV? Why or why not?

7 Can you tell if a person has HIV or AIDS by how he or she walks?

No. A person with HIV or AIDS can walk like any other person and display a variety of characteristics. Sometimes students will suggest that a person with AIDS will walk like he/she is sick. In this case, the person walks like he/she **feels** sick which is quite different than walking like he/she **is** HIV. Other people who feel sick due to different illnesses can walk like they feel sick, too.

8 Do some people with HIV or AIDS get treated differently than other people? When can special treatment be good? When can it be bad?

9 What is discrimination?

10 What is a stereotype?

11 How should people treat individuals with HIV infection or AIDS?

12 What does it mean to walk in somebody else's shoes?

13 What is involved with walking like you're sad, proud or happy?

14 Are people with HIV infection or AIDS also able to walk like they're happy, sad or proud?

Yes. People with HIV or AIDS are people, not their disease.

15 What does it mean to "walk the talk" of HIV or AIDS prevention?

16 What was the purpose of this activity?

Lesson Extension & Assessment

1. In small groups, students create other respectful and non-threatening activities that could assist the class in addressing stereotypes or exploring discrimination.

2. Students research legal issues pertaining to discrimination against people with HIV or AIDS. Sample questions could include: Do schools still discriminate against people with HIV? What is the Americans with Disabilities Act and what does it say about HIV and AIDS? What are legal issues regarding confidentiality and HIV or AIDS status? Groups determine and execute their own presentation methods and styles to communicate their research findings. Display or present the research projects.

3. Students create art posters that communicate the message(s) from the Walk Like Activity. Display the posters.

4. Students present the Walk Like Activity to their families, at home. Each student writes a detailed description of the teaching experience as well as the family's reactions. Compare and contrast the experience of participating in the activity versus presenting it.

Acknowledgments

EveryBody™ has been made possible, in part, by the generous support of

The Elizabeth Glaser Pediatric AIDS Foundation
The John M. Lloyd Foundation
The Harris Foundation
Danny Kaye & Sylvia Fine Kaye Foundation

RAD Educational Programs is grateful for the unstinting efforts of those individuals and organizations listed below whose energy, expertise and wisdom have contributed profoundly to EveryBody's success.

EveryBody Review Committee

Silvia Barbera
Marvin Belzer, MD
Jim Gilchrest
Jennifer Lamont, MEd
Deborah Main, PhD
Judy Margolis, MD, MPH
Lynelle Thomas, MD
Susan Frelick Wooley, PhD, CHES
Joseph Woolston, MD

Fernwood Project Advisory Board

Jean Adnopoz, MPH
Marvin Belzer, MD
Marta Benitez
John Brett, PhD
Marlene Canter
Bob D'Alessandro, MS
Charles Deutsch, ScD
Trish Devine Karlin
Irving Harris
Fred Miggins
Liz Pava, JD, MBA
Marion Johnson Payne, MEd
Darlene R. Saunders
Jean Schultz, MS, CHES
George Stranahan, PhD

Brand Strategy and Creative Direction

FM Branding

Design

Margaret Mathers Graphic Design
Wajskol Associates
Jenna Goldberg

Name Development

Wilder Advertising

Publicity

Selby ink

Editorial

Ellen Kleiner

And...

Leslie Burkholder
Sherry Caloia, JD
Christopher Colucci
Susan DeLaurentis
Ariel Flores
Elizabeth Glaser
Judith Goldstein, PhD
Charles Goldstein, JD
Chris Jennison
Abby Lochhead, RNC
Lisa Robbiano, RN FNP-C
Joede Schoeberlein, M. Arch, AIA
Mirelle Schoeberlein
Raphael Schoeberlein
Fred Sherrill
Kim Spence, DO
Janis Spire
Susie Zeegan